The Bad Widow Guide to Life After Loss

Moving Through Grief to Live and Love Again

by
Alison Pena

Edited by Anne White
Book design by 100Covers.com

ISBN: 978-1-7377905-0-1

To my mom, Anne White.

There are no words. I love you, appreciate you and am inspired by you every day.

*"The new dawn blooms as we free it.
For there is always light if only we're brave enough
to see it, if only we're brave enough to be it."*

*Amanda Gorman
National Youth Poet Laureate*

TABLE OF CONTENTS

"But what is grief if not love persevering?"

Vision from 'WandaVision,'
Episode 8 in "Previously On"

FOREWORD

Loss is a natural part of life, a key component of the human experience. It is normal, something we all expect to feel at some point. Yet, nothing can really prepare you for it. Grief is devastating, especially the kind that follows one of the most crippling losses—the loss of a partner.

There's no wrong or right way to grieve. After a loss, that sadness will present itself in many different ways. It will appear in every emotion you can think of, and even some you don't. Yet, despite the fact that this very real emotion affects us so powerfully, there aren't many spaces where you're allowed to experience it safely.

The world we live in doesn't honor grief the way it should. The stigma that surrounds the experience is absurd, especially since grief is at the core of humanity. A grieving person is sooner ostracized than understood. At the Emotional Institute, I teach classes that give people a safe space to explore their emotions— including grief—in a way that helps them discover their beauty, as well as better understand themselves and others.

It was in one of these classes that I met the real Alison. She stepped into my classroom, looking very ordinary. Simple, in fact. But there was a depth in everything she did. As an expert on somatic emotional release, the breath is a key part of every lesson I teach. It was in one of these breathing exercises that I got my first hint of Alison's inner strength. She drew me in with her inhales. They were profound. It was as if each breath mattered to her, and she was intimately connected to each one, drinking in the energy around her. Throughout the lesson, Alison was present to everything in a way that was so raw and vulnerable it made me pause. I knew instantly that this was rare to see.

Yet, it was the pools of depth behind her eyes that struck me the most. It was clear that she was well acquainted with grief. She was so sober to every fiber of the sadness she was feeling. She allowed it to engulf her, confident that she would make it to the other side. It was truly breathtaking to see, like watching birth at every moment.

I'm profoundly grateful to have met Alison, even more so now that she's chosen to share her writings as a gift to you, the reader. The depth of the experiences she'll share with you, and her unique way of thinking of and experiencing grief will enrich your spirit. Alison has an innate curiosity and willingness to truly *go there* that makes for a rare kind of authenticity. She'll help you to discover every nuance of feeling and to experience the freedom that comes from being so intimately connected with your emotions.

Thinking back to our time together, I can say in complete certainty that Alison grieved fully. She took her time with it. She had such a relationship with her grief that it made me ask myself, "When have I ever dared to grieve like that?" It was raw. It was real. It was the kind of honesty you don't often see in adults.

Though Alison calls herself the Bad Widow, her work has brought this world an immeasurable amount of good. She has helped so many people move through grief to live and love again after a heartbreaking loss. I think of her as the ultimate guide on a journey such as this one—a trusted friend to lean into; she holds your hand while you experience the cornucopia of emotions that grief ignites within us.

The fact that you're reading this is proof that you are in the right place. *The Bad Widow Guide to Life After Loss* will help you to experience yourself—and your grief—in a way you never have before, to take an honest look at yourself and ask what next. If you're struggling with what lies ahead and how to navigate your life after a devastating loss, then this book will help you take a big, nourishing bite out of the life that is possible for you. Alison is the real deal. She will help you master the waves of emotion that come with loss—from grief and anger, to shame and loneliness. Every bit of it.

So get ready for a ride, because it's definitely going to be one. Strap on your seatbelt, put on your helmet and grab your tissues. When Alison opens up and lets us in, she does so in a way that allows us to see ourselves in a new light. By the end of this book, you'll come out on the other side into a life well-lived, because you're well-grieved.

Bernadette Pleasant

"If you gave someone your heart and they died, did they take it with them? Did you spend the rest of forever with a hole inside you that couldn't be filled?"

Jodi Picoult
<u>Nineteen Minutes</u>

Introduction

On September 10, 2016, my husband, David Beynon Pena, died in my arms at home, just the two of us. After being diagnosed with Stage 4 pancreatic cancer in 2015, he lived for 11 months, far beyond the typical lifespan of less than 6 months.

Toward the end, as he declined and needed oxygen 24/7, family, friends and doctors urged me to move him into hospital hospice. People kept telling me, "You can't handle it." Always a contrarian, I answered, "You have no idea what I can handle." At home alone was the ending we both wanted and I was willing to fight for it.

After David was diagnosed with Stage 4 pancreatic cancer, most of the doctors suggested he should slow down, do less, take it easy. But that advice made no sense to us. If time was short, we wanted to live full tilt boogie. Meanwhile, the unspoken message was, "Prepare to die." Put your affairs in order. Go to the lawyer if you don't have a will. Make a plan to deal with the cancer and chemo side effects. Brace yourselves for the heartbreaking prospect of David's getting weaker, losing hair and leaving me behind.

Instead, we decided to live and love every day fully until the last one. We reprioritized and removed toxic people and activities from our lives, as much as possible. We wrote out our bucket lists — his, mine and ours — posted them on the refrigerator, and began knocking off the most important items. We chose to do what we enjoyed with the people we loved most. After 25 years, a relationship can become about who's taking out the trash or making dinner. Expressing love becomes less important than handling the logistics of daily life. And so it was with us.

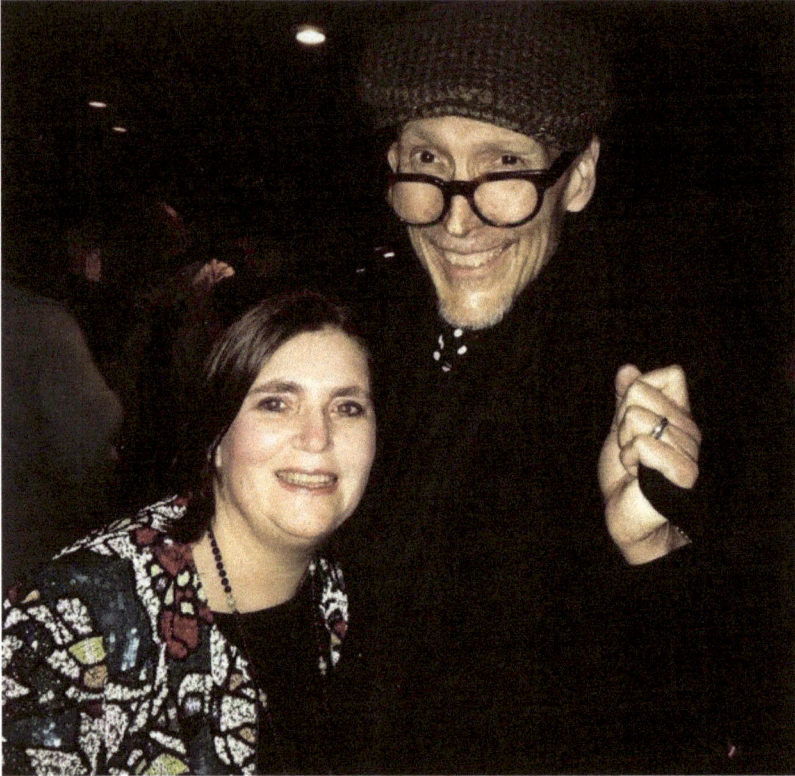

In March of 2016, David was undergoing chemo and getting thinner. But he was well enough to cheer me on at my first group cabaret show at The Duplex on 7th Avenue in NYC.

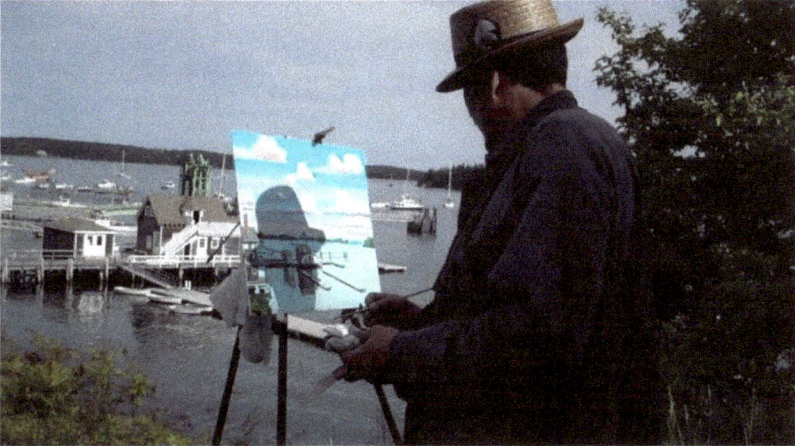

David Beynon Pena, before cancer upended our lives, painting a harbor scene on North Haven island, Penobscot Bay.

"We bereaved are not alone. We belong to the largest company in all the world — the company of those who have known suffering."

Helen Keller

Why I'm Writing This Book

Fighting for David's life those last 11 months and facing his death, David and I learned to live and love fearlessly. Those lessons turned out to be essential to my ability to reinvent my life when I became a widow.

Loss of a spouse or partner is heartbreaking, but we all experience losses that affect us deeply throughout our lives – from the death of a loved one to divorce, from loss of a job to failure of a business, from a health crisis to financial stress, from losing a pet to moving out of a longtime family home.

I'm writing this book to help others move more easily through the aftermath of their losses by sharing my experience and the strategies I developed, after David's death, to build a vibrant, expansive life that centers around what matters most to me. I also want to support people to grieve their losses, in whatever way feels true for them, as I did, in their own time, on their own terms, instead of reacting and responding to the expectations of others.

The Pandemic

In the last eighteen months, with so many losses due to Covid-19, the number of people suffering from mental, emotional and physical effects has skyrocketed. The pervasive, global impact of these losses is extensive.

- Not just deaths but inability to mourn together

- Not just lack of touch but fear of other people's lack of caring
- Missing out on celebrations of birthdays, anniversaries, graduations
- Loneliness, social distancing, isolation, aging
- Anxiety about how to stay safe and pay the bills
- Caregiving with inadequate support
- Social justice protests and destructive riots

Counting the Cost

The grief crisis that has engulfed so many people who suffered through these last eighteen months, due to the coronavirus pandemic, with record numbers of business failures and people losing their jobs, through no fault of their own, has had a global impact. Multiple interrelated crises, including cracks in our healthcare system, climate change and a partisan divide, have revealed systemic breakdowns we will be dealing with for years to come.

We all experience loss in our lifetime, so grieving is a universal experience. But we don't talk about it. We treat grief as an experience to be handled privately, rather than expressing it openly with family and friends. This lack of communication often leads to misunderstandings between a person who is grieving and those who care about them. This can damage even the closest connections as we lose trust in ourselves, our relationships and the world we live in, and end up feeling very much alone.

When I became a widow in 2016, I felt broken and was ashamed of my inability to 'just bounce back'. Some of my friends and family members treated me as if I might never recover. Others insisted that I needed to make major changes in my life, at a time when I was immobilized by the most devastating of changes, the loss of my husband of 25 years.

It impacted my confidence, my comfort level around people and my ability to be resourceful in solving issues in every area of my life. I reacted by pulling back, reducing my activities and interactions with other people.

It's normal to contract after loss, then integrate, learn, heal and expand again to live more fully. In fact, profound loss often gives us a deeper appreciation for life itself. But it was not until my longing for more joy got bigger than my fear of devastating pain that I was able to find a way to leverage my own innate resilience to take back my life.

I designed new strategies to move through the grieving process at my own pace and in my own way, refusing to be the kind of widow that societal expectations dictated I should be.

I've shared my Bad Widow coaching strategies for re-engaging, reinventing yourself and rebuilding your networks on many podcasts. This Bad Widow Guide is one of a series designed to offer you relatable stories and actionable resources for thriving on your own terms, in your own way, as I have done.

How Bad Widow Was Born

I chose to call myself Bad Widow because I know from experience that there is no one right way to grieve a heartbreaking loss, only yours. Despite the world's expectations of how a widow should act, every person's journey is different.

This book is designed to introduce you to my journey and the strategies I created to navigate the turbulent waters of loss, grieving and opening up to experience joy and love again. At the end of each chapter, there are insights and action steps to help you, the reader, chart your own path through your grief. My grief resilience coaching business is data-driven, personalized to solve each person's specific challenges.

Most of my clients come to me when their longing for more gets bigger than their fear. Once they decide they are heartbroken but not broken by their circumstances, we begin closing the gaps between their 'right now' reality and their deepest desires to live fully and joyfully again. Life is short. Are you ready to stop settling for less and live fearlessly?

Here is the story of the day my life as a widow began.

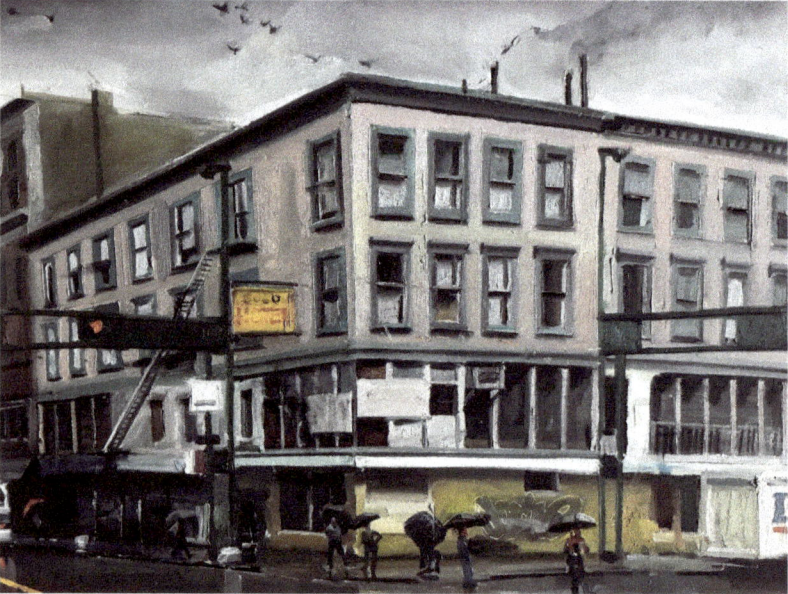

Umbrellas on a Rainy Day, NYC

Your Heart Beats in Me

Like the ley lines of my city,
Surges of energy pulse.
Like the beat of kettle drums,
Subway music calls.

Like tugboats on the East River,
Hauling barges home.
Like the homeless woman,
Feeding pigeons with found crumbs.

Like Times Square billboards,
Flickering lights and ads.
Like the New Year's ball drop,
To raucous cheers on a chilly night.

Like the touch of your hand,
On the skin of my face.
Like a whisper, there and gone,
Still, your heart beats in me.

Alison Pena

*"Death is a challenge. It tells us not to waste time.
It tells us to tell each other right now that
we love each other."*

Leo Buscaglia

CHAPTER 1

When Death Parted Us

I knew he was leaving that morning because I heard the theme song from 'Ghost'.

But David was anxious. He asked me: "What about my mom? What about my paintings? What about the studio? What about you?" I just kept answering, "Don't worry. I'll take care of everything." Holding back tears, I told him, "In a body, you need breath and love. When you leave a body, all you need is love. So whenever you're ready, go out on the love."

His head lay on my right shoulder, with my hands resting on the skin-covered bones of his rib cage. I tilted my head back so the tears dripping down my face would not hit his skin. By the end, he was 6' 3" and 146 lbs. Shortly afterwards, he took four long, slow breaths, and left me. Suddenly, after 25 years with this man, I was no longer a wife but a widow. The man I had hoped to grow old with was gone.

"Love takes off masks that we fear we cannot live without and know we cannot live within."

James Baldwin

CHAPTER 2

Diagnosis to Death –
Our Last Months Together

Life is short. Imagine if tomorrow was your last day. One day, it will be. For you or someone you love. That's the simple truth but we don't live that way.

For David and me, September 10th, 2016 was that last day. But we had no regrets, except that our time together was ending. We had learned how to live and love fearlessly, while we fought for his life and faced his death. What experiences would you regret missing out on if time ran out?

The Diagnosis

On October 12th, 2015, my husband David was diagnosed with Stage 4 pancreatic cancer. But this was not the first medical challenge we had faced together. Our marriage had been a roller coaster ride all along. Six weeks before the wedding, he was diagnosed as manic-depressive, then, a few years later, as diabetic, and finally with the cancer that ended his life.

On that Monday morning in October 2015, after a CAT scan the Friday before, the gastroenterologist called us in and told David, "It looks as if you have Stage 4 pancreatic cancer."

With his life expectancy now measured in months instead of years, we did not know how much longer we had together. The five-year survival rate for Stage 4 pancreatic cancer patients is 2.9%, so it was hard not to despair. But David and I decided to fight for his life, hoping we could win, that he might be one of the few who beat the odds.

After so many years, our marriage had become about logistics, with predictable routines, in a rut. With David's diagnosis, we realized that there was no time to waste.

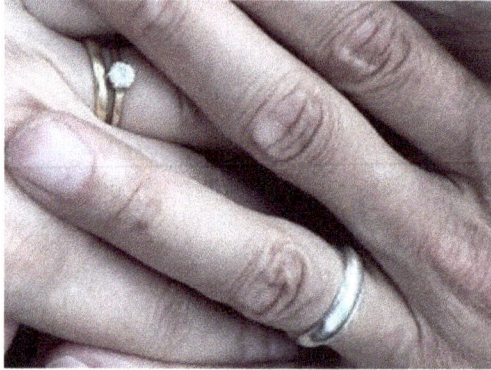

David and I took this photo of our linked hands a few weeks before he died in my arms at home

But how to make the most of that time, however long or short it turned out to be?

- How to live fully and fearlessly for however many days we had left together?
- How to thrive in the midst of our fear, grief and anger even in the face of death itself?
- How to sustain myself while caring for him, so that I would be able to recover again one day?

Pancreatic cancer was not anything we chose. It showed up and knocked us down, shattered our lives. The cancer was an inescapable reality, so we had limited options. First, the medical choices — which treatment to follow (he chose chemotherapy) and what doctors to work with. Who could we trust? And there were the choices about how we would live in the time remaining — whether to slow down and prepare to die or to live fully for the rest of his days, our days together.

We chose to commit wholeheartedly to what mattered most to each of us, and together, to live fully and love each other.

I started pushing David to do whatever he loved most, within the limits of his waning energy. This included enjoyable interactions and activities, not connected to work, which we tend to put off as nonessential. If he didn't love doing something, it got bumped. I also began participating in more activities I loved, including fulfilling a couple of 10-year-old bucket list items; in the months before David died, I spoke about my work at three big business networking conferences and sang in four group cabaret shows.

Coming Back to Yourself After a Loss

Everyone has moments when every decision turns out to be the 'right' one and every action gets perfect results. Every desire is answered, without even asking. This happens when we are doing what comes easy, in our natural zone of genius. But few people know how to access that place of thriving effortlessly. I found a way. The key lies in what I call the Affluence Code®.

Before life and cancer knocked us down, I spent years observing myself and other people, looking for the secret to living fully and joyfully. I discovered that everybody cares about three areas in life: work, relationships and community. And each person has one area they care about most deeply. Operating in that 'zone of genius' reduces struggle and leads to a more vibrant, successful and rewarding life.

The distinctions I created help my clients to thrive on their own terms, by figuring out what they care about first and foremost and choosing to focus on that. This leverages their natural way of operating in the world, their Affluence Code®.

I knew David needed to focus on his work to thrive. And my first priority was to contribute to my community. Understanding this was critical in anchoring us into who we were, even while facing heartbreaking circumstances. Trusting what I had learned and taught my clients enabled us to live fully and fearlessly until the end.

For both of us, relationships were our second priority. David loved to paint, play tennis and spend time with family and friends. An effortless extrovert who enjoyed parties, he was flamboyant and generous; he loved connecting with and encouraging people. So instead of slowing down, as the doctors advised, I created an environment where he was able to work and be around family and friends. I brought home his watercolor kit, brushes and easel and set them up in the living room. He finished his last commission there, on oxygen, two days before he died.

I also reached out to friends, encouraging them to come see him. Throughout his illness, we spent more time with people we loved the most and I'm convinced that made life worth living. And toward the end, I urged everyone to visit right away — or they would miss seeing him alive.

When we went in for checkups, bloodwork and chemo, his oncologist said, "Whatever you're doing, keep it up!"

Self Care

For my own wellbeing, it was important to remind myself that I was not just a caregiver fighting a losing battle, but also a woman, not just a wife whose husband was dying, but also an entrepreneur. And if I became a widow, I would need to create yet another role, rebuilding my life without him after 25 years together.

I began increasing my self-care and taking somatic healing classes to move all the feelings through my body as I was by his side for doctor's appointments, chemo treatments and ER visits. I tried to hide my grief at the changes in his body and the prospect of a future without him, while he tried to hide his fear, grief and anger at dying, which left us both lonely.

There were many heartbreaking moments...

- The day he lost his hair, eyebrows and eyelashes, riding a Citi Bike through the streets of New York, two days after starting chemo

- The nights he insisted on ushering in the theater after chemo treatments, even though the side effects made him throw up

- The day I chose to put my own self-care first and he said, "But I'm the one with cancer"

I wasn't the one who was sick, but I was profoundly impacted, my life turned upside down to care for him. I willingly set aside my usual activities and became his primary caregiver 24/7. But this created an impossible situation for me. As the person holding everything together, it would be bad for both of us if I fell apart. Yet, to stay whole myself, I needed to take time for my own self-care.

Because my first area of focus is community, part of self-care for me included serving others, even in the midst of my own pain and vulnerability. It's how I thrive myself.

I joined a cancer caregivers' support group and openly shared the journey David and I were on, posting on social media. This helped other caregivers and people with cancer feel seen and less alone. I also asked my community for a list of self-care practices to tap into when I was totally exhausted and couldn't think.

At home, I focused on creating a nurturing and loving environment, including designing a love meditation to comfort us when we were scared, angry or sad. And part of what sustained me was performing in two group cabaret shows, a longtime dream of mine.

Singing has always been a big part of my life. When I was a child, my family sang together. As an adult, I sang in a gospel choir for 10 years. And after David was diagnosed with cancer, I began singing regularly in cabaret shows, a practice I have continued since his death. My singing brought deep happiness to both of us. David was so proud of me. Four days before he died in my arms at home, he pushed me out the door to do my final cabaret show.

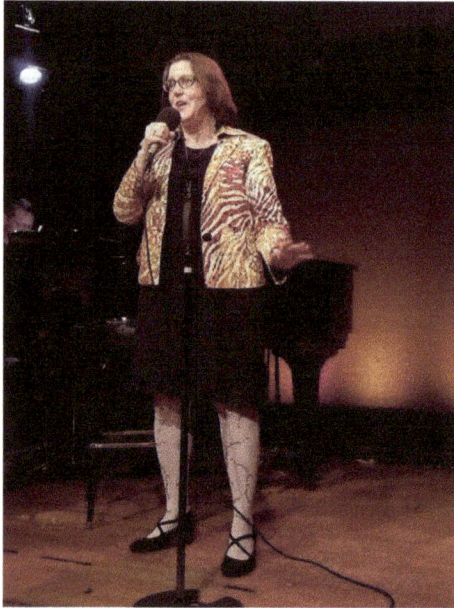

The songs I chose that evening reminded me that I was more than someone who was about to lose the man I loved for 25 years. Close to tears, I sang, *I Will Survive, Everybody Says Don't*, a rebellious song, and *The Secret of Happiness*, a song about how true happiness lives in the present.

David was 6' 3" and weighed 267 pounds when his cancer was diagnosed. At the end, he weighed just 146 pounds. I couldn't sit on his lap anymore or put weight on his body, because I would have crushed him. It was a heartbreaking time for both of us. But we made the most of it, finding new purpose and love in the midst of impending loss.

We just kept asking ourselves: "What truly matters? And if it matters, why not get to it?

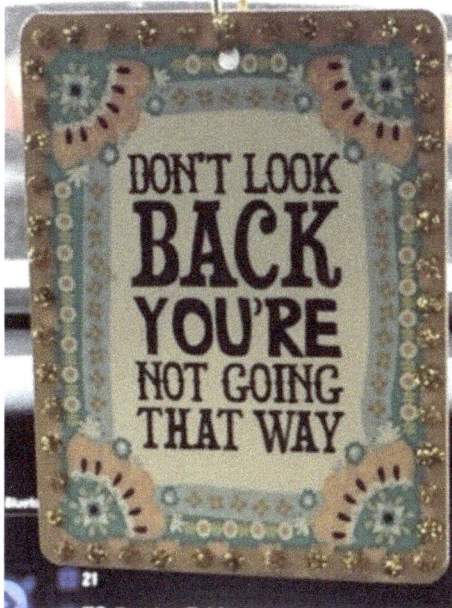

I saw this in an Uber I took to get to the first business networking event I attended after David died.

It was one baby step in the direction of taking back my life, even though being around so many people exhausted me.

Insights

People ask each other, "What would you do if today was the last day of your life?" as a hypothetical question. In fact, for all of us, one day will be our last. It's a simple truth we don't like to talk about.

Action Steps

1. Ask yourself, "What would I most regret not having said or done, if time ran out unexpectedly?"

2. Identify a conversation or action that is an urgent priority for you to complete before you die, whether it's taking steps to heal a relationship, pursue a passion project, embrace the work you were born to do, or _____ (fill in the blank with yours),

3. What is the first step you need to take immediately to accomplish your desired outcome? Begin with the end in mind, then build a bridge of sequential actions to take between start and end point to reach your goal.

If you are looking for grief support and tips, subscribe to my free Life After Grief newsletter, delivered to your inbox weekly. https://grief.beehiiv.com

To see more David Beynon Pena artworks for sale, go to https://chairish.com/shop/penafineart

"The best way out is always through."
Robert Frost

CHAPTER 3

Why Bad Widow?

Choosing to call myself Bad Widow was a turning point moment for me.

After David died, I felt broken, perhaps forever, and people treated me like I was. I didn't trust myself. I didn't know what I wanted and needed or how to begin climbing out of the depths of my grief and despair. And into that void, other people put their ideas about my needs, wants and desires. Everyone had their own beliefs about how I 'should' act as a widow, especially about the length, depth and intensity of my grieving process. But I wasn't getting the support I needed because people who loved me had no idea what to do differently.

This started to change once I started calling myself Bad Widow, a few months after David's death. As I began my journey back to living fully again, I realized I couldn't chart a path forward until I acknowledged that there was no going back and the future David and I had imagined would never come to pass.

Once I chose being resilient over being broken, and created Bad Widow, I was on my way. I began sharing the stark reality of what it feels like to lose the love of your life after 25 years. And I started to educate people on how to support me more effectively in my quest to heal and risk living fully again.

I told people how to ask better questions with a more limited timeframe. I couldn't answer "How are you?" But I could answer, "How are you today?" or "How are you right now?"

This was especially important when I faced an anniversary or other event where I knew I might cry. I reassured people in advance, saying, "My emotions are all over the place. But even if I cry, I'm not broken. I'm OK. You don't have to worry about me." People relaxed. The alternative to my clear communication was that they often said or did something stupid.

I get a lot of pushback on the name 'Bad Widow'. "But you're a nice widow, a good widow." I'm a Bad Widow because I decided I could no longer just go along, as a good widow would, saying "Thank you. That's very kind, I appreciate it." A bad widow like me speaks up and says, "This doesn't work. And this would work better."

As a Bad Widow, I tapped into my own resilience to solve the breakdowns I experienced myself. I now serve my clients with the solutions I created, supporting them to re-engage in life, reinvent themselves and rebuild their networks.

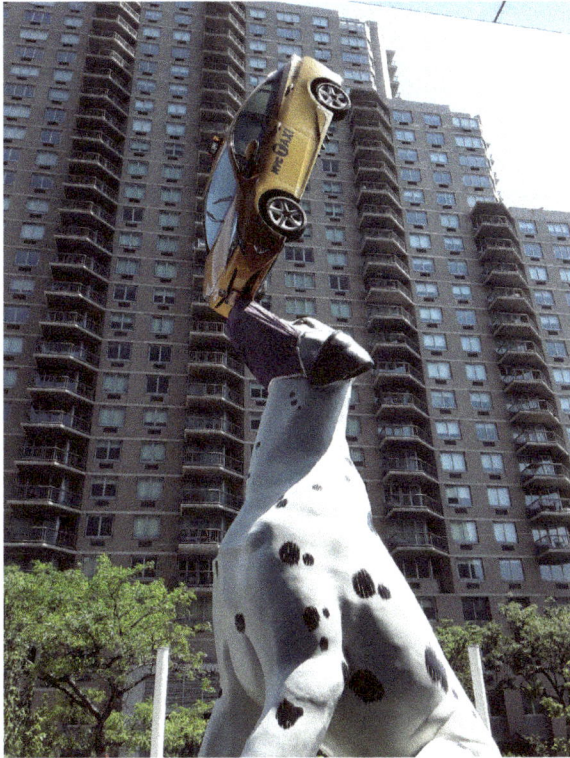

Dalmatian statue in front of Hassenfeld Children's Hospital at NYU Langone, wearing a violet mask to stay safe. This is how I felt too, balancing a life I no longer understood like this taxi, feeling utterly alone, yet still standing..

"The reality is that you will grieve forever. You will not get over the loss of a loved one; you will learn to live with it. You will heal and you will rebuild yourself around the loss you have suffered. You will be whole again but you will never be the same. Nor should you be the same nor would you want to."

Elisabeth Kubler-Ross

CHAPTER 4

Surviving My First Years Without Him

For me, the first year was all grief. The second year, I could go from zero to full-on rage in five seconds, for no reason.

When a loved one is given a terminal diagnosis, people tell you to prepare for the end — prepare a will, talk about finances and last wishes. You can do all that, even determine to live fearlessly in the remaining time together, as we did. But you can't prepare for the moment when the person you loved is gone, and you'll never see or touch them again. There's no way to prepare for that.

What happens to people after a heartbreaking loss?

- They feel broken
- Numb, just existing
- Overwhelmed by fear, grief, anger and shame
- They experience inconsistent energy levels
- Inability to focus
- Memory gaps

These breakdowns negatively impact work, relationships, health, time and money. How do you get back on track when life turns into a struggle just to make it through the day?

Right after David died in my arms, friends of his called with requests that seemed completely oblivious to my overwhelming loss and pain. There was the friend who was scheduled to visit him on the day he died. When I called to tell him not to come, that it was too late, he asked: "Oh, can I come over and say goodbye?"

And I couldn't speak.

Or the artist who called two days later: "Would you mind saving a few of Dave's shirts for me to wear while I paint so I can remember him? I am feeling so bad." Again, I couldn't believe it, and responded: "No, I'm sorry. NO!"

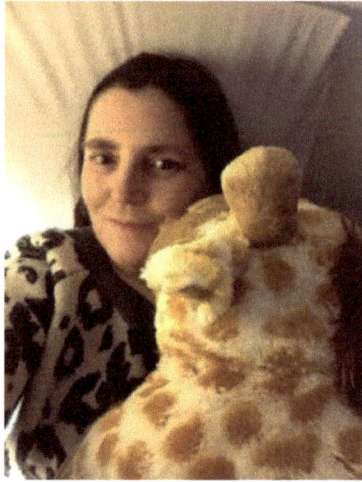

Sleeping badly made my inability to focus, memory gaps and flagging energy worse. So I got a Girow (giraffe/cow): huggable, big enough to comfort me, and feel safe enough to sleep.

That first year, I would lie in bed mostly asleep with a visceral memory of David's warmth at my back. Then I woke up and remembered he was dead. Every day. I was sleeping two to four hours a night. People suggested that I take a nap. And I answered, "I can't wake up to that raw, wrenching grief more than once a day."

Every day, I wouldn't get up until I found a reason to stay alive. I had to think of something to give me joy before I could leave the warmth of my solitary bed. I started with baby steps like… take a hot bath, call a friend, arrange to meet someone, take a walk, go to a movie, read a book, write a poem. Otherwise, I wasn't sure I was going to make it.

It felt like I was going crazy, as my short-term memory deserted me. I remember getting in the shower one morning, and when I got out, I was sure I had taken my shower, except I was still dry. In my memory, I was certain I had showered.

If I had a fleeting thought that I was hungry, I had five seconds to get to the kitchen before I forgot again. I put baskets of power bars all around the apartment so I would have a visual cue to eat and not have to rely on my spotty memory.

My best friend put up a small sign by the door that said, "Keys, phone, purse, shoes." One time, I got halfway down the block, on my way to an appointment, before I realized I was wearing my slippers, instead of shoes. I only noticed because my heels got cold from the wind blowing on them.

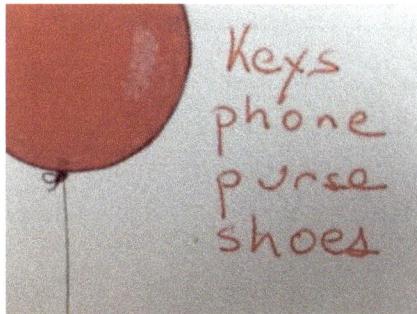

My best friend made this for me to put by the door when I was forgetting all the simple, obvious things I needed to go out.

She also made me a sign that said, 'NO,' about honoring my own experience and refusing to be with people or participate in activities which drained me.

At my lowest point, I thought I might be better off dead. I had hospice drugs from my husband's last days in the refrigerator. Making a deliberate choice not to take that path each day was a triumph for me. Widows, especially those without children, think about or commit suicide often enough in the first three months after losing a spouse that it has a name – the widowhood effect.

Holidays, parties and events were particularly hard without David:

- September 10, 2016, 10:10 am, the day he died
- October 1st, 2016, his memorial service
- October 5th, our 20th wedding anniversary
- November 24th, Thanksgiving
- December 21st, his 57th birthday
- December 25th, Christmas
- December 31st, New Year's Eve

Family and friends braced themselves for me to burst into tears. They would say, "Oh, I'm so sorry. I didn't mean to make you cry." It's uncomfortable to be around overwhelming feelings, especially grief or rage, because people think they should be able to fix it and don't know what to say. Whenever someone asked me, "What can I do for you?" I thought, "Give me back my husband!" When I couldn't bear it, I turned away or lashed out. And they left, sometimes forever.

Even, "How are you?" was impossible for me to answer. I wanted to say, "How do you think I am?!" I was looking at a wasteland of grief, the future I dreamed of, gone. I discovered that people had no clue how to deal with me. Unwittingly, they often said or did the wrong thing.

To right myself, I began to write and share poetry and stories about how I was feeling. They were raw and real — a profound act of self-expression and self-care. Writing gave me a way to ground myself when I felt like I was going crazy. This mostly true ghost story was written in the first six months after David died.

A Ghost Story

David hadn't traveled with Abigail before, not really, since he died in September. He stayed in the apartment mostly, turning the TV on in the next room, answering her questions with Pandora songs on her cell phone, flickering lights and blowing out candles.

This weekend, Abigail was headed upstate to Cooperstown, New York on the bus, a 5-hour ride, for a writing intensive. At the rest stop, the bus driver banged on the 1-person bathroom door, shouting, "Is your husband on the bus?"

Abigail started weeping, "No, he's not on the bus. He's dead." This was the moment she knew that, although David was definitely dead, he was apparently also on the bus. She wasn't sure he could do that, how long the leash of his ability to travel stretched. In fact, Abigail had hoped he was tethered to the apartment and New York City. Honestly, she needed a break. He was a very active and communicative ghost.

After checking into The Rose & Thistle B & B, a classic Victorian, painted pink of course, Sue, the innkeeper, showed her up to her huge attic room, bright and airy with skylights and a claw-footed tub. Sue's tongue rattled along like a runaway train going off the tracks.

Abigail stopped listening the moment she passed the wedding dress on a tailor's female dress form, halfway up the winding stairs to her room. Sue was a widow too, and acted as if they were the same, except Abigail's loss was months old and Sue's was years ago. Not the same at all. All she wanted was to collapse on the queen-sized bed, gaze at the sky through the skylight and stop. Just stop.

The workshop started that night, meeting at the home of our writing instructor Leslie, for introductions, a homemade farm-to-table meal together, and a start to writing. After Abigail entered, Leslie and her three students, Elizabeth, Terry and Abigail, settled on the plush, tan couch and armchairs with mugs of hot tea, pens and paper.

Abigail took the chair opposite the teacher, across the low wooden table, caddy corner to the other students. She was still struggling with too many people, more than just herself. And touch. Abigail feared that she would shatter if someone touched her; she could barely stay in her skin, so she avoided getting too close to people. David had not shown himself since she got to Cooperstown and Abigail was glad.

There was a ceiling light over the living room table with four bulbs, which started flickering as soon as she sat down. "Oh no, I replaced the bulbs before you arrived. I'll have to ask Christopher, my husband, to check them again, I guess," said Leslie.

"Don't bother," Abigail muttered, "It's David." Communicating with electronics was easy for him — lights, cell phones and TV. Abigail seldom talked of ghosts. She didn't want to be called crazy.

"Oh, OK. Good to know," Leslie responded. David stilled the lights and they began to write.

Abigail wept with abandon through the movement class, held in loving arms. She wrote what she wanted to let go of, added a few of David's ashes from a vial she carried in her purse, and sent the twist of white paper adrift down a nearby stream.

At the museum, they gained inspiration, wrote wild, dark and passionate. And drew pictures, David's gift, not hers. Abigail was best at dark. Making art brought pain. A walk in the countryside past horses growing their winter coats grounded her with every step on the frozen, rutted road.

Back in the living room with chamomile tea, everyone settled into their usual seats to share the day's writing. Before sharing hers, Abigail mumbled, "Mine isn't going to be any good." And the light went out over her head. All the rest, three of them, shone clear and strong. She took a deep breath in, the sob underneath, closed her eyes. Everyone waited, no words.

Opening her eyes, tears tracking silent down her cheeks, as her breath sighed out again, Abigail answered, "OK, David, I'll stop being mean to myself". And the fourth bulb lit and shone as brightly as all the rest.

Moving Forward

Grieving is a profoundly individual journey. Writing righted me and helped me make sense of the world, as I figured out how to live on without David.

After he died, I no longer knew who I was, where I was going, what to do next. And there were so many practical things to handle in that first year.

Most urgent was finances.

David wanted his paintings to sustain me after he was gone. His mother talked about how he left a million dollars' worth of art. But I had no idea how to turn paintings and drawings into cash to pay the bills. It was all I had left of him and I was savagely attached to every piece. If a collector or dealer quibbled over the price of a painting, I got really angry and refused to sell.

Earning income by selling his art or getting a job were both beyond me. I was barely able to function, much less work as a coach, proofreader or editor, as I had in the past. I had stopped opening mail, so full of medical bills for so many months, and almost had the electric, phone and internet turned off several times. I was grateful to be supported by family and friends, including financially, but I was reluctant to ask.

It felt shameful to be so incapacitated, unsure when (or if) I would recover and become self-sufficient again. I let my situation get to emergency status before I reached out for financial support, acting like a victim and making it hard for people to say, "No."

To my deepest regret, during this period of time, I damaged some important relationships, which I am still working to heal.

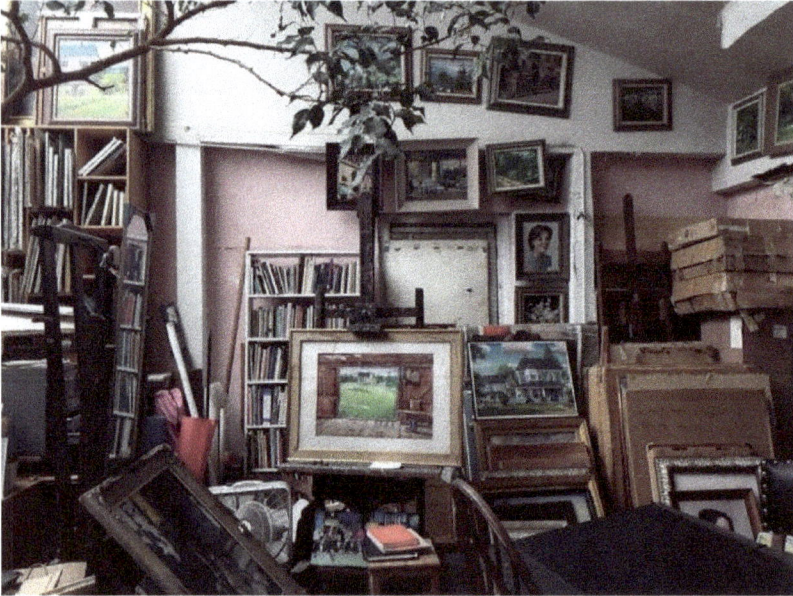

A corner of David's penthouse studio on Union Square, NYC

In September 2016, when David passed away, we lived in a one-bedroom apartment in midtown Manhattan. David also had a 500-square-foot studio in a prime location on Union Square, where he worked for more than 30 years. He left me a legacy of hundreds of paintings and his deathbed wish was for me to hang on to the studio for as long as I could. This was unsustainable, as our two incomes shrank to just mine, still with two rents to pay, plus all the other bills, including medical expenses not covered by insurance, even after his death. Barely able to care for myself, it was overwhelming.

His studio, the biggest and best in the building, had a soaring 24' ceiling, skylights, north light — and the highest rent. It was crammed with paintings, easels, bookshelves, flat files, books, art materials, frames and paintings. I knew the paintings would be the hardest to deal with, because they carried so much emotional weight. Every time I went into the studio, I was hit by the pungent smell of clove oil, which he used to keep the oil paint malleable. And I would burst into tears.

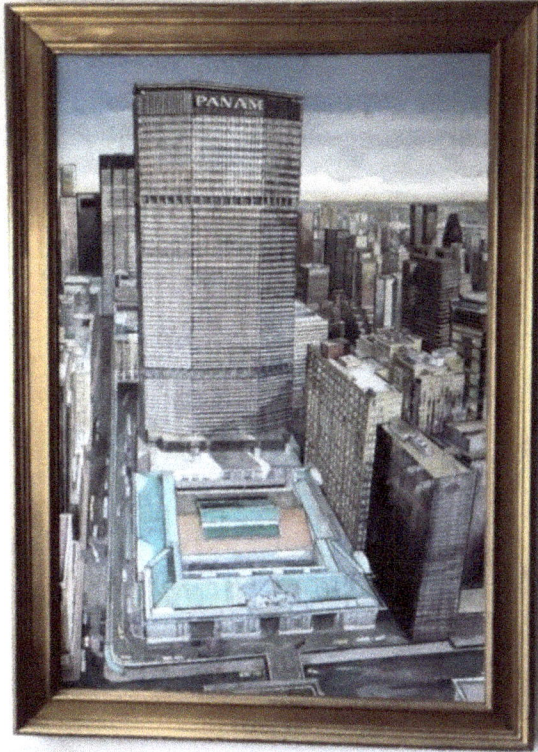

The Pan Am building, 1984

Making Hard Choices

Deciding what to keep and what to give away was excruciatingly painful. At first I tried to do it alone, but gratefully accepted when David's artist friend Eric from down the hall offered to help me break down bookshelves and decide which of his art books, paint brushes, easels, frames and painting supplies to sell or give away.

Then there was the question of what to do with the enormous trunk of painting materials that David took with him when he painted weddings and parties. I wanted to give it to another event painter, but anything unopened still held the smells I associated with David's body and his art. I couldn't open the trunk alone, so I asked Eric, who stood with me through all the ups and downs of clearing the studio, to come witness its opening and help me assess what was inside.

Most difficult of all was the task of sorting through all the paintings to determine what to do with them, which to keep and which to let go. This process was further complicated by David's practice of stapling three, five and seven paintings on top of each other on one set of stretcher bars. I had to uncover each painting to the last layer and decide what to do with each one. Some days, I wound up with my fingers bleeding after pulling out staples for hours. It was a fascinating process that said so much about who David was, an endless discovery, layer by layer. It was also dismaying to uncover so many hidden paintings at a time when the thought of letting go of even one broke my heart. There were already so many to cope with.

The culling process was brutal, but I had no choice. I couldn't keep or move it all. I didn't know what David would want me to do and he wasn't here anymore to ask. It made me so angry! I didn't have money to rent a storage facility, so the paintings were going to have to come home with me and I needed to reduce their number. If I couldn't sell or place a painting, it had to be destroyed because I didn't want unfinished David Beynon Pena original art out in the world, devaluing the rest of his legacy. He never threw out any painting, watercolor or drawing, so there were many that were unfinished. I covered up his signature with an oversized sharpie before stuffing the rejected canvases into big, black trash bags.

I was making good progress getting rid of stuff when building management threatened to fine me for creating too much trash.

I was stuck, so much to throw out with no money to pay for dumpsters or movers, and management trying to get me out ASAP. I even found them a perfect tenant to take over the lease, but they wanted to terminate David's lease so they could hike the rent.

Bringing David's Studio Home

Eventually, I brought all the paintings, books, flat files, easels, bookshelves and painting equipment home to my apartment, designing a ritual to step myself through the process.

I loaded furniture, paintings, books and supplies on moving dollies and a hand truck and began walking them home from 16th Street and Union Square to 30th Street and 2nd Avenue. As I balanced his flat files, filled with works on paper and loose canvases draped on top, people stopped me along the way, asking questions. I began telling the stories behind David's paintings to complete strangers.

The evening I walked home, pushing David's John Christen Johansen's 8' foot tall standing easel, that was given to him by his close friend and mentor, the world-famous portrait painter, Everett Raymond Kinstler, I was stopped again and again by curious bystanders.

Over the course of several months, I discovered exactly how uneven the sidewalks of New York City were, how helpful or unhelpful people could be when I was struggling up a curb, how dolly wheels sometimes have a mind of their own. I found that if everything wasn't balanced just right, the dolly yawed all over the street, pulling me this way and that. I hung frames over my shoulders, while I carried Players Club crystal glasses in my hands. It was an experience between weeping and joy, so exhausting my legs and heart hurt.

One day, when I was worn out, taking my last run of the day, a man saw me at the corner of 16th Street and 2nd Avenue, struggling with a load that kept falling apart. He immediately turned around and pushed my heavy load all the way home, refusing anything but my thanks. He said, "Anyone would have done the same." I called him an angel. His kind act restored my faith in the goodness of people.

Finally, an Uber and van finished the moving job and I turned over David's studio. Everything I was keeping from his 500-square-foot studio was in my 850-square-foot apartment. You do the math. I had a 12-inch passage to make my way through the living room, things on either side stacked and ready to fall on me at any moment. Every time I walked through the door, I was swamped with memories, seeing all the paintings helter-skelter and remembering when and where he painted each one, while I sat beside him reading a stack of books.

Selling His Legacy of Art – From Tears to Joy

What was I going to do with all these paintings when the sight of them made me cry, the prospect of selling them overwhelmed me and the thought of letting them go seemed impossible? David was excited to leave me so much art, hoping I could support myself by selling his paintings. He also left a book draft that he wanted me to get published, along with 50 sketchbooks. It was all too much, at a time when I could barely get out of bed.

His artist friends asked, "How are you going to curate his work?" I thought, "What about MY life and MY dreams?" I needed to figure out how to take care of his legacy without giving up on my own.

Slowly, I began to take back my apartment and my life. I hung 50 + paintings on the walls. Laying two bookshelves on their sides, I created racks for stretched and framed paintings. Other paintings live in the office, living room, dining room and bedroom, and the books fill my office bookshelves to the last inch. With an eye to the future, the most saleable paintings, watercolors and drawings have been imperfectly photographed and placed on his online gallery website, and on a few other websites that sell art.

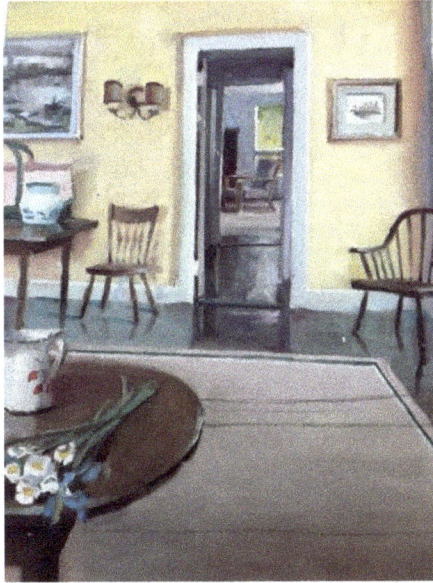

Summer House Dining Room Interior

At first, there were only a few painful sales, partly because I was uncertain how to price the paintings, where to show them, and reluctant to let them go. But by 2019, I was ready to release more of them to new homes to be enjoyed by others. I had a gallery show in Maine, where some of the paintings were sold. I offered my nephews art to decorate their dorm rooms at college. Now, I am working with an art dealer to honor David's intention for the sales of his art to support me and fund my dreams.

It has taken me close to five years to feel joy instead of heart-break as his paintings, watercolors and drawings are sold to new collectors to be appreciated on other people's walls. And I am finally ready to reclaim space for me and my boyfriend, Wayne, by reducing the sheer volume of David's work that now dominates our apartment, physically, visually and emotionally.

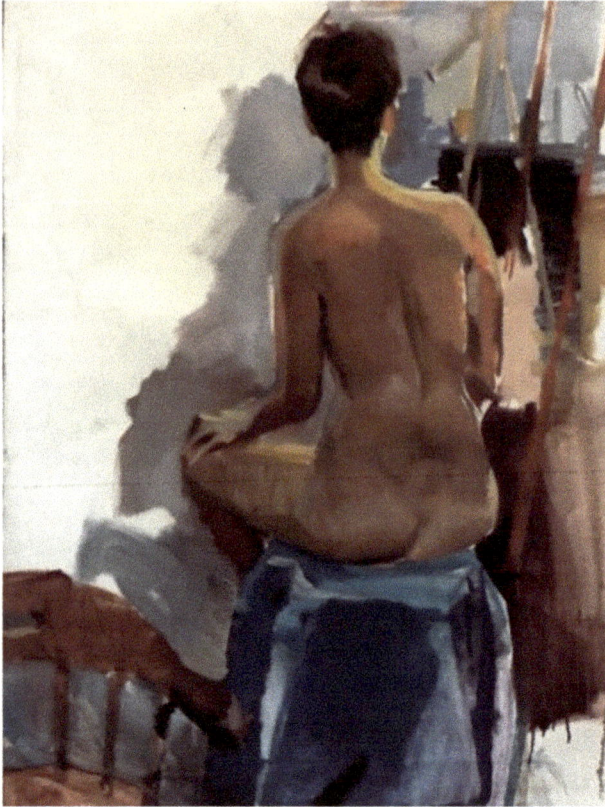

Insights and Action Steps
Handling Overwhelming Feelings
and Letting Go of Stuff

Insights

Feelings, especially out-of-control, overwhelming feelings, make people uncomfortable. They disturb the peace of both the person experiencing them and the ones witnessing that fear, grief, anger or shame. Holidays and celebrations are especially difficult, as the person grieving may be out-of-sync with everyone else, may even burst into tears unexpectedly.

Stuff left behind by a loved one may also be charged with emotion, especially if it taps the senses in some way. A favorite album or song (sound), the smell of my husband's paint cut with clove oil (smell) and his paintings hanging (sight), food from a special place (taste), a shirt he used to wear all the time (touch). Any of these types of memories can provoke unexpected, unwelcome feelings.

Action Steps

Plan ahead. Think about what you will do if tears threaten or if you actually burst into tears unexpectedly in a public place – at work, at a party or in the street. Remember that for most people who care about you, their instinctual reaction will be to try to fix it somehow. They want you to be OK. Their solution may or may not be helpful to you.

  1. There are several possible options:

      a) Let people know in advance that this might happen, how you want to be treated if it does and that you are OK

47

b) Excuse yourself and leave the room for a private place

c) Cry if you need to and don't worry about what other people think

2. When you are going through stuff which has emotional meaning for you, and deciding what to keep and what to let go of, make sure to invite a close friend to be there if you think that might help. Often, telling the story of the item to someone else provides a moment of lightness, even laughter, while tackling a difficult task.

If you are looking for grief support and tips, subscribe to my free Life After Grief newsletter, delivered to your inbox weekly. https://grief.beehiiv.com

To see more David Beynon Pena artworks for sale, go to https://chairish.com/shop/penafineart

One of David's most classic nude drawings. Being a widow for me was often like being stripped bare and remaking myself from scratch.

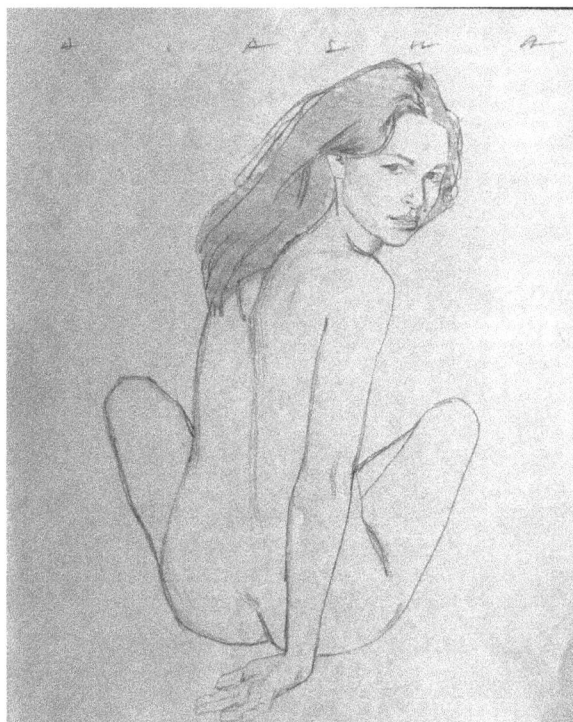

"We do spiritual ceremonies as human beings in order to create a safe resting place for our most complicated feelings of joy or trauma, so that we don't have to haul those feelings around with us forever, weighing us down. We all need such places of ritual safekeeping."

Elizabeth Gilbert
Eat, Pray, Love

CHAPTER 5
The Importance of Rituals

Rituals are part of everyone's lives. They mark the passage of time and events in our lives, happy and sad — marriages, funerals, anniversaries, birthdays. Some birthdays and events have more weight than others, like sweet 16, high school graduation at 18, seen as an adult at 21, a quarter-century at 25, half-century at 50, retirement at 65, 75, 100. There are holidays like Christmas, Hanukah and Kwanzaa, and events like bachelor parties, baby showers and retirement parties.

In order to move forward, after David died, I created my own rituals for aspects of grieving which were especially hard for me – letting go of the studio and paintings, clearing space for his legacy and my new life as a widow, and deciding what to do about our wedding rings and David's ashes.

Wedding Rings

One of the most important rituals of marriage is the exchanging of rings, "With this ring, I thee wed." David asked my father for my hand in marriage because he was old-fashioned that way. My Dad answered, "Yes, of course, but why are you asking me instead of her?!" My engagement ring was cubic zirconia although few people knew. It was as beautiful to me as a diamond and affordable for an artist. Giving me that ring allowed him to save face with my family.

The wedding ring I put on David's finger when we married was not the one he was wearing when he died. David went through three wedding rings in our 20 years of marriage. I thought it was funny. As long as he wore one, I didn't care. Wearing our rings said we belonged to each other in the eyes of the world, no trespassing.

For 20 years, we wore our wedding rings. But what now, after his death? When the minister, David's mom and my mom left the apartment that last day, I took off my engagement ring and put it in a gray pottery bowl my brother made.

Then I removed David's ring and found out that he had put a little piece of white sticky tape inside, to keep it from sliding off as he got thinner. I placed his wedding ring, including the tape, on my bureau in front of a card I which says, "You are made of stars." I got it for him before he died. David was gone forever and this ritual act marked his leaving my life and our marriage.

The last time I wore my wedding ring was at David's memorial service on October 1st. I sat in the left-hand pew with my family, listening to the service I had planned, tears streaming down my face, completely numb as people shook my hand at the reception and offered their condolences for my loss.

After the memorial service, I took the tape off David's ring and put it with mine on a gold chain around my neck. The two rings hung against my collarbone, my ring nestled inside of his, close and tight, and, if I spun mine inside, they linked like planets, circling.

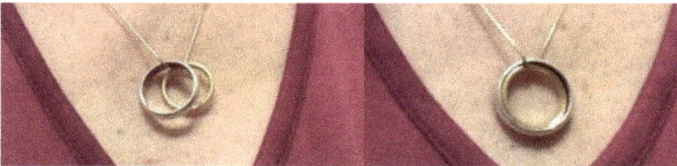

Our wedding rings, circling like planets and nestled together.

Letting Go

I wore both those rings, his and mine, until I began longing to date again. Our rings and his ashes were the tangible reminders of our 25 years together. To make space for the possibility of new love, I knew had to let them go. On July 1st, 2018, as I prepared to go on my first Bumble date, I put our wedding rings on their chain in the gray ceramic jar with my engagement ring. After that, each time I went on a date, allowed a touch, dared a kiss, tsunami waves of grief rose up. I learned to let myself be, even as my ring finger is still indented with the mark of where my wedding ring sat for 20 years.

In my first year as a widow, it was impossible to believe David was gone. I could hardly stand to be touched and even a spark of desire felt like a betrayal of him. Over 25 years, my skin had grown used to his, the weight of his arm around my waist, and no other hand in mine or kiss on my lips felt right.

Gradually, I came to recognize that these new feelings simply meant I was making a choice to open up to the possibility of love again. If I allowed David to occupy all the space in my heart, there would be no room for anyone else. I worried that my dates might feel that living up to a beloved, dead husband, who would never make another mistake with me, was an impossible bar to reach. And that wasn't okay.

I don't want to go back, but sometimes the sadness rises and I miss David, even as I love Wayne, my boyfriend whom I live with now. The taking off of rings in a gradual ritual allowed me to see that I was moving forward. This was a choice I could make at a time when life had knocked me sideways and I had no control over so many areas of my life.

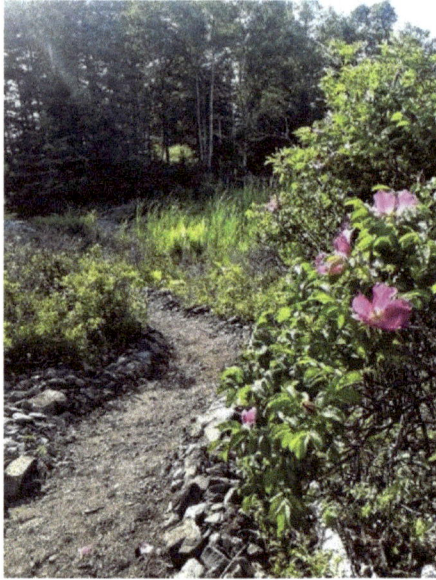

I scattered David's ashes on this path at Wooster Cove in Maine

After Ashes Go to Ashes

Nobody wants to talk about death and what happens afterwards. But with David's stage 4 pancreatic cancer diagnosis, we had to talk about what to do with his body after he died. A grave and headstone, coffin and worms. I had no car to visit a cemetery. An urn or box, fire and ashes. A funeral or memorial service. How fast or slow did the service need to happen?

It was an emotional, heartbreaking conversation because this decision acknowledged we were planning for the likelihood that he would die. David wanted to be cremated because it was easier and cheaper. I wanted him to be cremated so I could scatter his ashes in Maine and other places he loved. Joyce, his mother, assumed he would be buried because, in her world, "That's what everybody does." When David told her he planned to be cremated, she said, "Oh no! You didn't discuss that with me."

When a person dies, there are so many questions. The decision that he would be cremated was one he and I made together, while he was alive. I found the idea of ashes more palatable than a body in a grave and was comforted by their portability. I liked the idea of spreading his ashes all over the world so he could be everywhere. But still I wondered…

Would David care if he sat in a porcelain urn on a mantel or was scattered to the winds? Would keeping his ashes be a deterrent, an omnipresent relic of past love getting in the way of future love? Human dust with more meaning than regular dust. I was reluctant to touch the ashes.

The ritual I developed to release his ashes helped to comfort me and honor him. It also amused me and allowed me to move forward.

David died in my arms at home on September 10th, 2016 at 10:10 am. I didn't even call the funeral home to come get him until 1 pm. I straightened his legs and arms on the bed so the attendants wouldn't have to do it after he got stiff and cold. When they arrived at 5 pm, I couldn't watch, so my mother did while I hid in the bathroom and wept. They put his body in a black body bag and took him to New Jersey to be cremated. Two weeks later, someone from the crematorium hand delivered this huge, rectangular, robin-blue box to my door and I had to sign for it. Inside there was a plastic bag with a massive amount of ashes.

I had no idea a human being would transform into so many ashes. I had no idea where to put them. I had no idea if they were sacred or simple dust. I wondered if the medical port in his chest that delivered the chemo or the stent in his lower intestines survived the flames.

I knew I didn't want them in the bedroom. I wasn't sleeping well anyway. I didn't want them in the living room for others to see. They were personal. I wanted the ashes to comfort me and I didn't know if that was even possible.

What I did know was that I wanted to have him with me, so I looked around for a likely container, small enough to carry in my purse. I chose a vial which used to hold bath crystals, the perfect size. A guy from my bereavement group joked that the vial was the Beyond in Bed Bath and Beyond. David would have laughed himself silly, which made me smile.

Before the memorial service on October 1st, I spooned some of his ashes into a small, glass jar to give to Joyce, his mom. I also gave containers to David's cousins to scatter in Australia. Then I hid the robin-blue box with the rest of his ashes on the highest shelf in the corner of my office, out of sight but not out of mind.

Ashes are the last physical remnants of a person. But basically, they are dust. People have mixed feelings about ashes. I have mixed feelings. I wanted David cremated so he would be portable and I hated the idea of visiting a grave. Yet I was tentative about touching and handling them. They weren't something that could be spilled and swept up thoughtlessly or that I wanted to touch with my fingers. I barely breathed as I carefully funneled ashes into various containers. Even a strong puff of breath could make them fly away and be lost.

Every time I went out, I stuck my glass vial of ashes in my purse so I could carry him around with me, always. It had to be secured inside a plastic bag, just in case the cork stopper escaped. I could just imagine the horror of David scattered all over my purse. I also had just a few ashes in a tiny plastic pill container, to fit in a smaller purse.

I took him with me everywhere. Anyplace he loved, I loved, or I thought he would have loved in New York City, I scattered ashes.

I scattered his ashes on Sixth Avenue where he used to paint street portraits on the sidewalk in his 20s, telling me the stories of inviting passersby to sit in his chair for a sketch, "Just 15 minutes!", competing with the other artists for customers. I sprinkled just a few in the bushes and fountains outside the National Arts Club, The Players Club and the Salmagundi Club, where he was a member. I wanted his ashes to be in all the places he frequented when he was alive — near the Met, the Natural History Museum and throughout Central Park. As I walked, I dropped them. I even reached through the bars at Gramercy Park to dust a few ashes on the winter snow, where they blended in, only to see them rise, chalky white, on the brown earth in the spring.

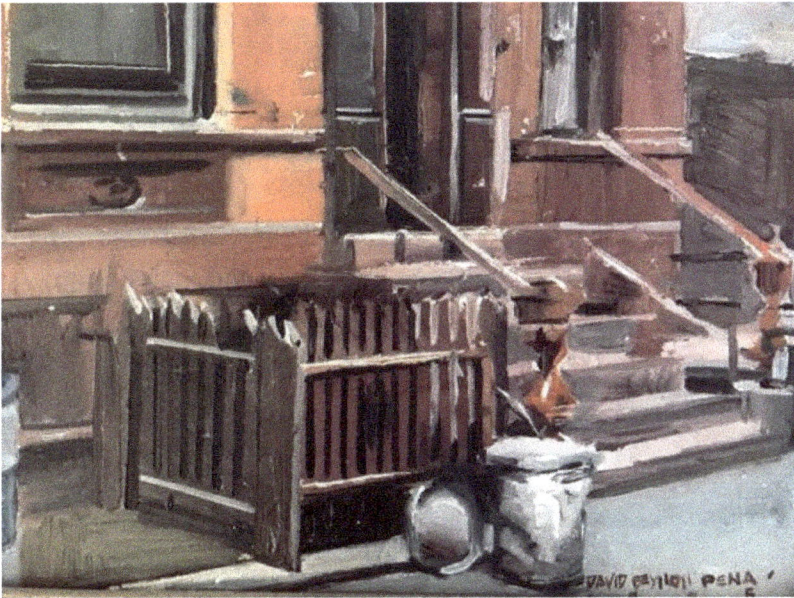

Ashcan School oil painting

It's illegal to scatter ashes in public spaces. So I would surreptitiously take the vial out of my purse, hide it in my hand, against the inside of my arm, and ease the cork out. Tipping it, I shook the ashes out of the glass vial like a salt shaker. When it got empty, I refilled it from the blue plastic container and headed off again. I was delighted by performing this nefarious act because David would have loved it.

I traveled with David's ashes too. I took them up to Old Chatham, NY to mingle under the tree with my father's ashes. I remember putting them close to the trunk. David always craved my father's approval and would have been happy to rest there with him.

When I went to France in 2017 to visit my friend, Makenna, at Julia Child's country cottage in France, they went with me there too. Transporting human remains across borders is illegal, so flying with David's ashes internationally was complicated. Nobody challenged me at the airport, but I was ready with my outrage and tears, just in case. I hid his ashes in a dry energy drink container. At the overnight layover in Morocco, I opened the hotel window, placed the ashes on the sill and watched them blow away on the breeze.

Once I arrived in France, I scattered ashes around the main house and cottage, up and down the paths and in the boles of trees, all over the property and nearby towns. I was glad to be there, but very sad not to have David with me. He would have loved to paint the pastoral landscape, the charming towns and the people. I think the place and people would have been delighted by him too, but leaving his ashes was the best I could do.

By 2018, David's ashes were widely spread in many places across the globe. But despite my best efforts, I still had this enormous robin-blue box of ashes, lurking in my office like a vulture. I was beginning to think about dating and opening up to love again, even though I was terrified. Looking at online dating apps, I realized that I had to let the rest of the ashes go to make space for new beginnings.

I knew I wanted to scatter his ashes in Maine, where we had our happiest moments, vacationing and painting. There was North Haven, where my grandparents had a house. I HAD to get to the path of stones we built from the beach to the dock at Wooster Cove. But new people now owned my grandparents' old property.

When we got there, they were reluctant to let us go down the path past the bulldozer that was clearing land around their new house. I persevered, clambering over the huge pile of earth, while my mother distracted the owners with conversation.

I was intent on having his ashes lie on land that had been in my mom's family since 1949, though we no longer owned it, and to pour them into the waves of Penobscot Bay, to become part of the ocean.

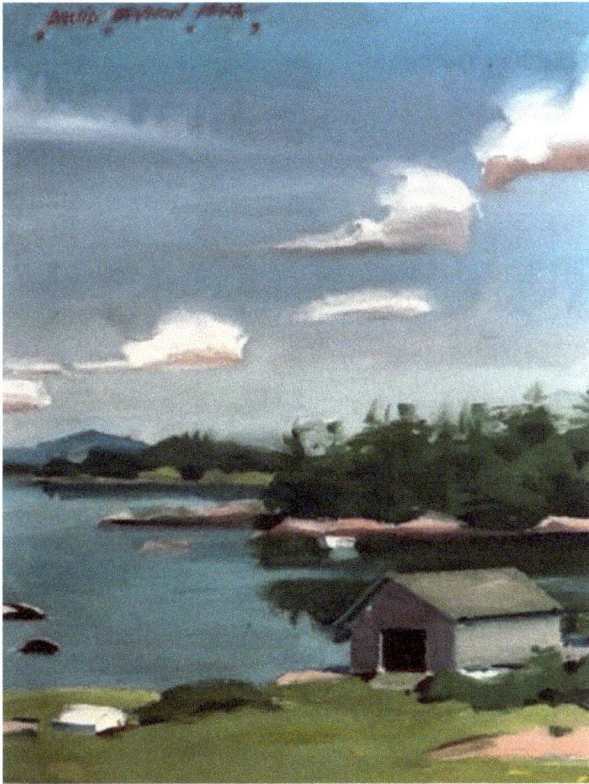

David Beynon Pena painting of Leadbetter Island

Then there was Leadbetter Island, bought by my father's parents way back in the 1930s, just 20 minutes away from North Haven by motorboat. For decades, I ran wild and free with my cousins on the island. When David came into my life in 1992, we began going to Leadbetter's together. Each summer for ten days, David painted two or three oil paintings or watercolors each day and hung them in the attic to dry, so he needed to be there too.

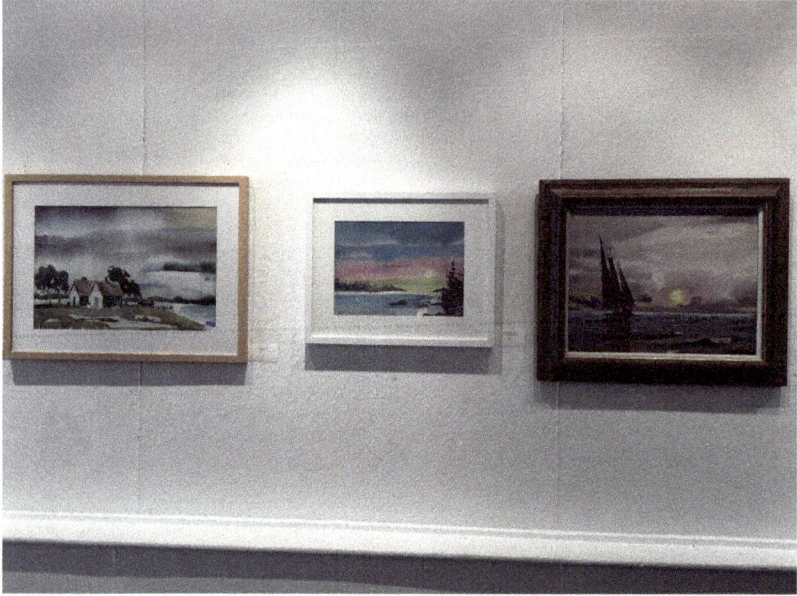

There were so many painful layers of letting go that summer of 2019 – selling paintings, seeing people who didn't know he was dead and scattering his ashes. After being unable to let go of any paintings, I had a gallery show of his work, with all the prep of framing, naming, packing and setting up beforehand and gallery sitting during the show. I was selling more of his paintings than ever before, telling the story of his last year every day as I gallery sat. It was heartbreaking and exhilarating. I had just three days after the show to finish my ritual of scattering his ashes.

I HAD to get to Leadbetter Island with the ashes because I had more memories with David there than anywhere else in the world, but we had no boat to get there. Larry, the caretaker, didn't call us back until the very last minute. I was desperate. It had to happen for me to move on. Finally, he returned the call with an, "Of course,

I can give you a ride out tomorrow on the Posy L.." That was the island boat named after my grandmother. It was our last day in Maine before the last of the ashes were finally scattered.

Back in NYC, on July 1st, 2018, I went on my first date since June 1992, when I met my husband, David Beynon Pena at a church retreat on the Delaware Water Gap. There is still a vial of ashes somewhere in the bookshelf, comforting but not looming, and not in the way of my new love.

Insights and Action Steps
How to Design Your Own Rituals

Insights

Beyond the rituals in our everyday life, it's helpful to develop rituals for those places where we get stuck or can't find the resources we need, so we have to create them ourselves. Grief is particularly rich ground for rituals because death is something we don't like to think about or talk about. Yet everyone dies.

Action Steps

1. Identify exactly where you are stuck. Is it feeling so numb that you forget to eat, drink or sleep? Is it releasing stuff or handling finances? Is it remembering to put on shoes before you walk out the door?

2. Think about what you could do that would solve that issue and implement it. That might mean putting up a sign by the door, attaching the missing habit to an easy working one or opening the mail as soon as it arrives.

3. Rituals have the meaning you give to them. I created many of mine to deal with uncomfortable situations, to let go of the past and to reassure myself that I was moving forward, even at times when I felt like I was standing still or wallowing in the past.

Maine holds lots of memories, happy and sad, with family,
friends and David.

When I imagine where I feel most peaceful,
Maine by the ocean is that for me.

This is so true for me, I specified in my Bumble profile that I prefer
rocky beaches to sandy ones.

Where is your peaceful, joyful place?

"We delight in the beauty of the butterfly, but rarely admit the changes it has gone through to achieve that beauty."

Maya Angelou

CHAPTER 6

Re-engage in the World

In 25 years together, David and I were wound around each other like vines.

Going through any loss, especially losing someone you love, hurts. Grieving after David's death, my world shrank. I had less energy to reach out to people, less interest in my usual activities. I was unable to focus. My memory was spotty. Uncontrollable thoughts, feelings and physical reactions impacted my relationships, my business, my health and my finances.

After a while, I really wanted to get back to work, see more friends and maybe even start dating. I just didn't know how. It was clear to me that I would not bounce back without a concerted effort to re-engage in the world again. I would need to step up and take action, even if it was only one small step at a time.

I looked at where I could begin to push out against my own fears even though my capacity was limited. I assessed the areas of my life — work, money, health and relationships — to decide where to start. What were my most urgent challenges? Which actions would make the biggest difference? I needed to start earning money again. So I chose to begin with work.

First, I needed to regain confidence in myself and my abilities by taking baby steps towards the life I wanted, tapping into my own resilience to build solid ground.

I began looking at where I could expand the boundaries I made to feel safe after David's death. Sideways, backwards or forward like a crab, every step provided a different perspective and opened up alternative pathways to move forward. The only thing that got me through the pain, grief, anger and shame, was wanting a bigger life.

Getting through the times we're living in right now requires a similar step-by-step approach, tapping into our innate resilience, past the guardrails we erected to stay safe and alive through the pandemic, back into the world after having our lives shaken up, even broken, without our consent.

Getting Back to Work

I was a medical editor and proofreader for decades, but after David's death, I couldn't remember a piece of content from one second to the next, much less from page 10 to page 250. I was unable to do any work I was qualified for. I had no energy to serve clients or work in an office. Yet, I needed to reconnect with people anyway, to do something to feel like a valuable, competent person again.

For my first job after I lost David, a widow friend who ran a Halloween pop-up shop hired me to work a 4-hour shift, four days a week. It was September and October of 2017, a year after David died, and a 'normal' work week was still beyond me. I could hang a costume on a hook and follow simple directions, often needing them repeated three times. And I was totally exhausted at the end of each 4-hour day.

I was not going to be hanging costumes on racks for the rest of my life but that Halloween pop-up shop job was to be a critical baby step for me. I just needed to start somewhere, to get back to working at any job. It was distressing not to be able to move forward from where I was before, but I couldn't. What was possible had to be enough. I was a very smart, capable person. Until suddenly, I wasn't.

I needed so much support after David died —emotional, financial, spiritual, physical — everything. I asked friends for financial help, and some said, "We are happy to help, but only if you are willing to be reasonable. Give up this consulting nonsense, move out of your apartment, go back to proofreading, and get a safe, secure job."

They did not understand that I could barely get out of bed. I had just cleared out my husband's 500-square foot studio and brought hundreds of paintings home. I had the attention span of a fruit fly and holes in my memory, which made it impossible to do the work I had done for over 20 years. The support would have been helpful, but the price was too high. I said, "Thanks, but no thanks."

When your whole world turns upside down after a loss, there's nothing solid to stand on. The advice and solutions other people suggest often feel wrong. The question in the uncertainty is, "How do you come back to relying on yourself and your own intuition as a foundation?"

Building Nets

Re-engaging in the world for me had a lot to do with solving for the breakdowns caused by the physical and emotional effects of my grief. By asking myself, again and again, "What's the solution for this breakdown?" I became my own North Star and eventually learned to come back to center effortlessly with strategies that worked. These breakdowns ranged from missing touch, to struggling to get projects done with no energy, from simply getting out of bed, to no longer trusting my memory, from being overwhelmed by emotions and memories, to forgetting to prioritize my own self-care. I call the solutions I designed 'nets'.

I needed human touch so much after David died. We had no children or pets. I had not understood how necessary that physical connection was for me to feel good, until it was gone. Once, when I was feeling depressed, I went downstairs to talk to the doorman for company. He asked, "Would you like a hug?" "Yes, that would be amazing!" I answered.

Studies have shown that people require 4 hugs a day for basic health, 8 hugs for wellness, and 12 hugs to thrive. I suffered deeply from lack of touch after David died. And during the pandemic, even one hug could put a life at risk, so we all became afraid of an essential part of our human connection.

No Energy, No Memory, No Focus

My energy levels fluctuated wildly and unpredictably. Some days, I had lots of energy, and other days, I had none. When I was exhausted, I was unable to think and my memory could not be trusted. So I wrote down everything I had to do for my consulting and tutoring work, taking care of my home and my health, including eating, drinking and exercise, self-care practices and fun. I wrote it all up on a whiteboard with Sharpies.

When I woke up in the morning, I checked in with myself, asking, "How much energy do I have today?" Then I chose options from the list on my whiteboard. If your energy is flagging or your tank is empty, it's really difficult to push on through. Writing down all the tasks and activities provided a net to move the action forward, slowly or fast, according to my energy level. Then, after completing any task, large or small, I'd celebrate like there was a circus in town, whether I just went for a walk or wrote six articles. Completion and celebration fueled me.

Some days, it was difficult to get out of bed. I would lie there and try to think of someone I could reach out to or some activity I could do which would bring me joy. After David died, joy was the least accessible emotion because it brought up grief at the same time. I had to learn to be grateful for moments of joy, even when I was deeply sad. There was also a deep-seated fear that letting go of fear, grief and anger meant betraying David, even forgetting my love for him. Yet, our loved ones would never choose for us to live without joy.

As for work, I was a former medical editor and proofreader who kept losing track of information and time. I might lose 10 minutes, one minute or a week. I felt like I was going crazy. This created a profound distrust of my body and mind, especially my memory, which lasts to this day. When I sang in a cabaret show in 2019, I was so afraid that I struggled to remember words I had practiced over and over, and was ashamed to crash and burn on one of my songs. I am now working to rebuild my lost trust in myself, a long-haul effect of my grief.

Too Many Out-of-Control Feelings

With my emotions all over the place, at first, I was distressed and embarrassed by my feelings of fear, grief, anger and shame. It was not until I acknowledged that these feelings were a reasonable response to David's death that I was able to reach out for help and move forward. I had to remind myself, "This doesn't mean there's something wrong with me. It means I'm grieving or angry that my husband left me here." I literally shouted at the sky at David, "You have it easy! You don't have to find a way to go on alone."

One evening I was so distraught, I couldn't go home. My husband's paintings and memories were everywhere, a constant reminder of what I had lost. So I went to dinner and a movie to calm myself.

I realized I needed friends who would be there for me at times like this. The following day, I made a list of five people I trusted. I asked each of them if I could call them up and come over if

I found myself in bad shape, even if it was 2 am. I only used it once. My friend, Stephanie, gave me tea. I rested on the couch as the activities of her home went on around me.

I knew I needed community and hugs but did not want to be treated as if I was broken. It was at Singers Space, an open mic in New York City, that I connected with people who would fill that need, a family of my heart. One evening, I cried for 30 songs out of 35. Afterwards, friends came over, hugged me and allowed me to be sad without trying to fix me. If this is you too, find a community that will support you as you are, and embrace the possibility of being happy again. Allow enjoyment and laughter to open up your world, even in the midst of tears.

Planning for Tears

Beyond my safe, open mic community, I designed strategies to handle unexpected tears in any situation. Tears simply mean you're sad. Yet too often, if someone is crying, overwhelmed or heartbroken, people say, "Just push on through. Get control of yourself." It's uncomfortable and upsetting for them to be unable to help, so they want the tears to just stop. But suppressing feelings impacts mood, energy, mind and body. Unexpressed emotions can get stuck in the body and cause serious health issues, if ignored.

Responding to a friend or stranger who asks about your tears, you can say, "Thank you so much for caring. I am okay. It's just been a rough day." They might offer a Kleenex or say, "Is there anything I can do?" Then you have the option to ask for what you actually need, for example, "Can you sit here with me?"

One of the most challenging and important places to handle emotions appropriately is at work. Blowing up at your boss or bursting into tears in a meeting can damage a career. I learned that proactive acts of self-care would buffer me when going into a difficult conversation or a challenging meeting. Sometimes it's critical to bank extra energy for stressful times. Self-care provides the essential reserves to get through tiring interactions with toxic people or unpleasant, obligatory activities.

The Importance of Self Care in Hard Times

My friends came through with a list of over 100 specific self-care ideas for me to tap into if I was exhausted and at zero capacity. When I was depleted, I could just choose one. Self-care and self-expression activities expanded my capacity to be more emotionally balanced and effective.

What do you do for self-care and self-expression? Here are 10 of mine.

1. Sing or read poetry at open mics
2. Walk in nature
3. Make art
4. Blow bubbles
5. Dance or move my body
6. Listen to music
7. Hang out with friends
8. Play with crystals
9. Travel globally
10. Visit museums

As adults, we often skip self-care as we juggle too many personal and professional appointments, projects and activities, thinking it has to be expensive or take a lot of time. When I felt stuck, I chose practices to move emotions through my body proactively. The somatic healing dance workshops I took with Bernadette Pleasant of the Emotional Institute were especially effective. Singing was mandatory, as it allowed my heart to heal and open again. I trusted my body to choose the 'right' activity.

One of the most valuable skills to master in stressful times is the ability to be present in your body — learning how to breathe, how to move, how to dance or sing. I created a way to do this using my five senses and focusing on my immediate experience. If you look at a tree and examine the bark up close, there's no room for anything else. If you smell a lemon with your eyes closed, you are focused in the present. And listening to music is a common, fast way to move emotions through your body.

There are also so many sounds in nature that can help you connect with your body. I took a conch shell and held it up to my ear, so I could listen to the ocean. It pulled me out of my seemingly endless grief and fear of the future back into living. I also use vibration to bring myself back to embodied, with music, drumming and singing bowls. Sound shifts the cells. If I can get myself into the present, I feel alive.

Insights and Action Steps
for Re-engagement

Insights

After any loss, as human beings, we contract our world, see fewer people and participate in fewer activities, to heal ourselves from our grief and pain. Depending on how long this takes, from days to years, eventually we want a bigger world again. My clients come to me when their longing for more gets bigger than their fear. It doesn't happen automatically. It requires bravery and making new choices. And it's much easier with support.

Action Steps

1. Figure out your Affluence Code®. What makes you feel most like yourself — when you focus on your work, your relationships or your community? Do more of what lies in your zone of genius, the things that are easy for you, to center yourself. We make better choices when we are grounded and it's easier to stay grounded when we're focused on what matters most to us.

2. Review all the areas of your life (whatever they are for you) to assess whether you are thriving — with your work, relationships, health, money and time. Fortunately, all of these are interconnected, so any action will shift one or more of the others. This is wonderful news when you are in thriving mode, terrible when you are in survival mode. Choose the area you plan to start with. There is no right or wrong answer.

3. Where to begin? Pick the area that's easiest with minimal emotional attachment (low-hanging fruit which provides encouraging progress) or pick the most difficult area (once done, you no longer dread dealing with it).

If you are looking for grief support and tips, subscribe to my free Life After Grief newsletter, delivered to your inbox weekly. https://grief.beehiiv.com

To see more David Beynon Pena artworks for sale, go to https://chairish.com/shop/penafineart

All artworks shown in this book are David Beynon Pena originals, which can be found on this website and others.

"Life isn't about finding yourself.
It is about creating yourself."

George Bernard Shaw

CHAPTER 7

Reinvent Yourself

In the 25 years we were together, David and I shared dreams and made plans, assuming we would love each other forever and grow old together. At 10:10 am on September 10, 2016, his life ended early. After he died, my future alone was unpredictable and uncertain. Time sometimes went fast and sometimes slow. Memories shifted around and I felt ungrounded, even crazy.

When a person experiences a heartbreaking loss, they often say, "I want my old life back." But that's impossible. After a loss, you're not the same person. You can't have your old life back. To acknowledge that reality, I created this definition: 'Loss is the death of a future imagined or co-created that will never come to pass'. This takes all the blame, shame and guilt out of the experience. It's just a fact. Accepting that reality grounded me so I could begin to reinvent myself and my life.

The first requirement was to get clear about who I was now, what I wanted, who I wanted to be around and how I wanted to participate in the world. Grieving and reinventing myself also revealed a greater appreciation for life and what truly matters to me now.

Sounds easy, right? It isn't.

David and I had been together as a couple for close to half my life. One of the main ways I identified myself was as his wife. None of us is the same person we were a minute ago, let alone after a losing a spouse or partner. If we continue looking at our life and priorities from before, we may be headed in the wrong direction. The major disruptions we experience after a loss actually provide an opportunity to take a real look and ask, "Is this the life I want for myself now and in the future?" If not, change direction. But how?

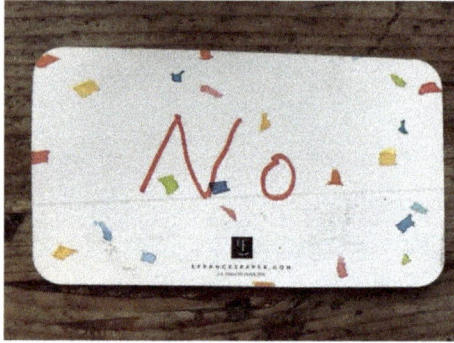

This sign was designed to remind me that I could say, 'No,' without guilt, to people and activities. And 'Yes,' once I figured out what I did want my life to be.

Making Distinctions to Map a New Path

The problem was that I no longer knew who I was without David or who and what I liked or disliked. Before I could reinvent myself, I had to get clear on what it meant for me to be an individual, not part of a couple, a widow, not a wife. With my new, unasked-for autonomy, I needed to figure out which of the choices I made over the years were mine, which were ours as a couple and which were David's alone.

That required asking better questions:

1. How, when you feel broken, can you find your way back to whole?

2. How can you trust your mind and body again?

3. How can you grow your capacity to make decisions and take action alone?

4. What markers can you set up to show progress in moving forward when time is slippery?

5. How can you ask for what you want, specifically and clearly, so that you get it?

To start back to feeling whole again, I had to do what I do best, lean into serving my community. In January 2017, four months after David's death, I started my https://BadWidow.com blog, speaking from the middle of the messy grief experience I was going through. None of the overwhelming feelings were under my control. The blog was visceral and raw, but it was also healing, both for me and for those who tuned in, a way for me to be vulnerable, sharing authentically and having it reflected back.

I couldn't find anyone speaking from that place where I found myself. Yet I was sure I wasn't the only one and discovered I was right, when other people who had suffered losses began writing to me privately.

Any loss changes the trajectory of your life, as priorities and opportunities shift. Moving on doesn't mean you're jettisoning everything you were. Your past will always be a part of you. Owning who you were, who you are, and who you will be can help carry you forward into your new life. It was hard for me to see that, especially right after David died.

I struggled to connect with people, keep appointments and work an 8-hour day. I couldn't trust my own mind and body, couldn't focus and remember stuff. I was afraid I might miss something important or let someone down, including myself. Even today, I don't fully trust myself, fearful that those memory gaps and panic attacks that occurred in the first year after David died, might return. Now I'm aware it may still happen occasionally, but I'm taking baby steps to ease my fear and rebuild trust in myself.

Losing Trust in Myself

I was an extremely competent person, a leader people looked up to. I knew how to build strong personal and professional relationships and make new ones. I made decisions and took effective action quite quickly. After losing David, I was no longer confident or competent and I found being around most people utterly exhausting.

My first action to take back my confidence was taking that job at the Halloween pop-up store just to be around people, doing work. I used to be able to do more but I had to start somewhere and build from there.

After a loss, time becomes slippery. The activities, relationships and interactions which usually anchor us in time, like going to school or the office and hanging out with friends, are gone. So we step out of the normal stream of time. This means a person who's grieving is out of sync with the rest of the world. Tasks or activities that used to be easy for them, no longer are, which can be confusing for colleagues who assume they will bounce back to 'normal' sooner or later.

Grief after losing a spouse has an assumed time limit of about a year. After that, people expect you to be ready to move on. It's common to hear, "You really need to get back to work" or "It's time for you to start dating again," accompanied by introductions to potential dates."

Other losses, like a job, a business, a home, a divorce, a pet, a health or financial crisis, are allowed an even shorter grieving period. Then we drag that unexpressed grief into our next relationships and opportunities, where it colors what we do in the future.

At the beginning, I couldn't trust myself to remember appointments, so they went in my calendar the moment I made them. I couldn't create goals any distance in the future, so I set up interim steps and celebrated each one. These actions helped me see that I was moving forward, even if my progress was slow.

Asking More Powerfully

Before losing David, I was reluctant to ask for anything because I assumed people would feel pressure to say "Yes," even if they didn't want to. I worried about owing them a debt I could never repay. Afterwards, I learned that many people wanted to help me, but just didn't know what to say or do. They would offer help: "Let me know what I can do for you?" And I didn't know how to answer.

People who have experienced the death of a loved one, or any heartbreaking loss, don't know what to ask for. I've heard from many widows and widowers that they want people to just 'know' what they need without being told. Yet, that makes no sense. Neither the grieving person nor those who want to support them get what they truly need and desire.

Clarity is a superpower. People wanted to give me everything I needed but they didn't know what it was. If I wasn't clear, they did not take action. The only way to get what I wanted and needed was to ask specifically, so they could not get it wrong.

These are my three steps to provide better support to a grieving person:

1. Ask what's going on and listen to what they share, without judgment.

2. Based on what they tell you, offer to help them with something specific.

3. If they agree, execute on your offer of help, asking for guidance as needed.

If you can get clear about what they actually need, take the initiative and act. It's a huge relief, because a person who's suffered a loss can't easily articulate what they need. But it's a delicate balance; they also don't want their autonomy ignored and their boundaries breached.

As an entrepreneur, I couldn't afford to be paralyzed for too long. I had to find a way to trust myself and map out my time more effectively. With clarity, life made more sense and I was able to learn very quickly how to expand and become more productive again.

Reducing my options was essential, especially when my attention span was short. I learned how to look out at the landscape of possibilities and screen out the ones which weren't right for me. This clarified what I actually wanted and narrowed down the millions of opportunities out there so I could decide, quickly and easily, what I needed most, and ask for it. Agility and speed are superpowers for any entrepreneur.

An Inspiring Story About Asking and Receiving

In March 2017, I experienced a powerful example of how being clear works when my landlord called and asked, "Where's the rent?"

My family helped me with rent after my husband died because I was barely able to function. So I said, "Remember, it's taken care of."

And she responded, "No. That ended in February. It's the 23rd of March."

I had no idea where the rent was coming from. I knew I would figure it out, but I was shocked. I sat down and wrote a blog post called, "Grief Brain and Bills."

At the end, I offered this advice: "If you have a friend who's afflicted with grief brain like me, here's what to do: 1) Have a conversation with them and listen to what they say. Do not ask, "What can I do for you?" because they don't know; 2) Offer to do something they need, based on what they shared; and 3) If they agree, follow through and get it done.

After I posted the blog, I still needed to figure out how to pay the rent. Within 30 minutes — and it still brings me to tears — my freshman college roommate, who I'd not seen since the last class reunion, responded on Facebook, "I'll pay your March rent."

Stunned, I answered, "I live in New York City, so feel free to back out." But she refused, saying, "No. Give me your landlord's name and address and I'll send it tomorrow."

I kept saying, "You are incredible. Thank you so much!" And she responded, "I just did what you said in your blog post."

It was such a lesson. I was clear about what I needed, the rent paid for March. She read what I wrote and offered to take action to answer my greatest need.

My responsibility was to figure out who I was, what I liked and disliked, and what support I truly needed, so I could make specific requests. I began making distinctions, asking myself, "Do I like this or that?". I started with, "Let me try this. No, that's not really my thing. Let me try that instead."

I began to look at what was important to me now as I reshaped my life on my own. Couples often compromise, especially in the beginning, each telling themselves, "I'm going do what he/she wants, because we're newly in love."

How many of my choices were shaped, early on, by what my husband liked, then set in stone over 25 years? For example, I loved open mics, but my husband, David, wasn't interested. Gradually, I stopped going. In those last 11 months, he encouraged me to sing in public again, even perform in four cabaret shows, and take back that joyous experience.

After he died, I began singing again and participating actively in the open mics I loved. I also started sharing original poetry as well, a new form of self-expression for me.

Reinvention means reprioritizing and putting time and energy towards your own new priorities. The key to making progress is to play, experiment and ask lots of questions. I made a game of it, making distinctions as fast as I could, because the future I was building was mine alone, not the one I'd lost with David by my side.

As David's widow, I am a different person than I was as his wife. I can look at my past and the choices I made, but my loss provided me an opportunity to reassess my life from a new perspective and decide if I am on the right path with work, health, relationships, money and how I spend my time.

One of the biggest challenges for me relates to David's massive inventory of paintings. How do I take care of his lifetime legacy of art, but not sacrifice my life's work for his? How can I carve out space for myself to live and love again?"

Stepping out and being willing to take risks was another area I struggled with. Having contracted my world, I wasn't sure if I could trust my instincts, so everything felt risky.

First for Women Photo Shoot

By February 2020, I was ready to begin expanding again, when an amazing opportunity came my way through my friend, Bernadette Pleasant. I was asked to do an article in 'First for Women' on how I used her somatic healing movement workshops to help heal my emotional turmoil. And I said "Yes!"

Then I waited and waited, not sure if it would really happen. Finally, in June, the magazine called and said, "It's on." — my first major media print opportunity!

I pictured it going differently. I hoped I'd be able to get a haircut, have my makeup done and lose a little weight, to look thinner for the photos. That's not how it went. With New York City at the epicenter of the pandemic in March and April, hairdressers had just opened up for business again and I couldn't get an appointment anywhere. Usually, the magazine provided a hair and makeup person but there was too much liability this time.

Unfamiliar with makeup application, my friend, Maurya Sullivan, offered to show me how to do it myself from Boston on Facetime. She walked me through every step of putting on my makeup, face to eyes to cheekbones to mouth, as I sat in front of a mirror 400 miles away and modeled each look. I don't know what I would have done without her.

Then there was the photoshoot itself. As I awkwardly demonstrated the somatic healing dance moves I learned in Bernadette Pleasant's movement workshops, and the magazine's photographer clicked away, I thoroughly entertained families, children and nannies in Central Park.

The First for Women article turned into a 2-page spread with four photos of me, published in September 2020. Friends all over the country started contacting me to tell me they had seen it. Not what I imagined, but the risk, ready or not, was worth it.

Knowing that life is short, I've become unwilling to compromise on speaking my truth. This happens a lot, not an unusual side effect for people after they suffer a loss. I've also gained clarity on my goals and priorities for the future.

I call myself Bad Widow because I challenge assumptions about how we grieve and support those who grieve, both at work and personally. I'm now designing my life's work, knowing it will include:

1. grief resilience coaching, focused on healing grief-driven personal and professional relationship breakdowns after loss

2. writing and publishing bestselling books, and

3. selling David's amazing legacy of art.

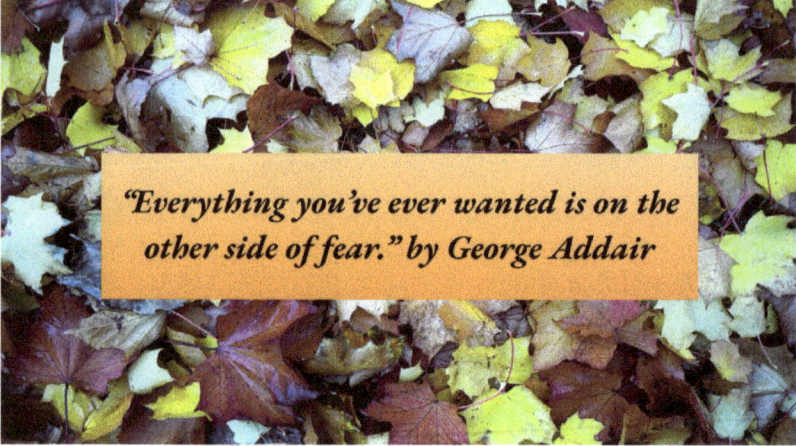

"Everything you've ever wanted is on the other side of fear." by George Addair

Insights

Reinvention begins with the realization that you can't go back, either to the person you were or to the life you had before your loss. Accepting that reality and looking forward instead of back for answers, is the start to rediscovering who you are, recalibrating your priorities and resetting your path into the future.

Action Steps

1. Accept that the past is history, you are a different person and your priorities may have changed. Loss shakes up lives and makes us look at what truly matters now and in the future.

2. Review the path you were on and the priorities that led you there. Consider any seismic shifts caused by your experience of loss. See if any of your priorities have changed and if those changes point you in new directions. If so, explore them.

3. Find out who you are and who and what you like and dislike. Discard your historical assumptions and experiment with new and old activities. Play is one of the fastest ways back to joy. Self-care (whatever that means to you) is one of the quickest ways to expand your capacity and feel whole again.

If you are looking for grief support and tips, subscribe to my free Life After Grief newsletter, delivered to your inbox weekly. https://grief.beehiiv.com

To see more David Beynon Pena artworks for sale, go to https://chairish.com/shop/penafineart

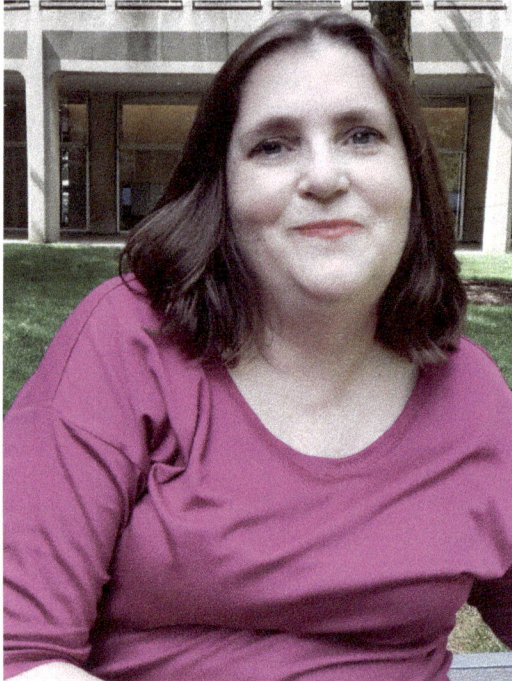

Ready, sort of, for my First for Women photo shoot. I chose the shirts I wore and got tips on what makeup to buy with a survey on Facebook., Maurya showed me how to apply it virtually, as I sat on the bedroom floor in front of a mirror.

"We aren't ruins. We are the rebuilding, the remaking, the revivals, the constant reincarnation of ourselves."

Nikita Gill

CHAPTER 8
Rebuild Your Networks

One of the biggest casualties of grieving a loss is losing relationships with people we counted on for support, as they disappear from our lives after a death or divorce, job loss or business failure. After David's death, I was hard to be around, especially when those who loved me felt helpless to do anything to help me.

People stepped up, or stepped back and stepped out when I was 'too much' or my grieving went on for 'too long'. If they couldn't handle their discomfort when I cried or raged about my situation, they left. Eventually, I started teaching people that they were not responsible for easing my pain, and my tears and anger didn't mean I was broken.

I discovered that there's a fictional time limit for how long people are allowed to grieve. After 25 years with David, it was a year. Then everyone moved on, except me. I was still grieving. I wound up with huge holes in my networks, at a time when I needed support more than ever. When David was alive, he always had my back. When he was gone, I needed my network to fill those holes, but it wasn't designed to provide me with that level of support.

It takes inner resilience to step back into life again. And net-works of support who are able and willing to provide necessary resources. Some people were easy for me to be around and others were hard. I identified two tiers of people — the ones who were energetically easy and those who were toxic — needy, over-helpful or insistent on telling me what I should do. As a protective measure, I stepped back from the toxic people for a while, the ones who would say, "I can do this for you, but only if you agree to do what I think is best." The people who were easy just let me be. If I said, "This is what's going on and I just need you to listen," they would do what I asked, without question.

I began to think about networks in a different way, realizing they permeate every aspect of our lives. They aren't just for business referrals or for improving our social life. Recognizing that any big change, especially losing a loved one, automatically impacts our relationships, I designed a strategy to look at my personal and professional networks, see where the holes were, and begin proactively filling them in. What if our networks could deliver on our dreams?

Typically, people fall out of our lives and we wait for someone else to show up by default. What if, instead, we curated our networks by design?

If you know where you're going, then you can determine who you're going to need along the way and when you get there. Once I identified my natural abilities and top priorities in life — "my zone of genius" — using the Affluence Code®, I was able to begin setting goals and expanding the relationships I would need for the future I was creating. And I began looking proactively for people who could deliver on my dreams.

One of my favorite quotes is, "Leap, and the net will appear," by an anonymous author. People will be your net if you allow them to be and show them how. When you are hurting, they are there. When you are on your way to everything you ever wanted, they celebrate with you.

How to Get What You Need to Thrive

Family and friends want to give us what we need, yet we are often afraid to ask, making our requests in a tentative way. Sometimes we ask for something so big that the person can't possibly deliver, so they don't even try. Or we ask for something so small that it doesn't make our own heart sing, much less inspire the person we're asking.

People want you to thrive and come back stronger. They want to give you more than the bare minimum you need to survive. And with six degrees of separation, someone out there knows exactly who to connect you with to realize your goals and make your dreams come true. Think of your networks as the key to unlock the resources you need.

When someone is grieving, they are often reluctant to ask for what they need because they look at interactions like a balance sheet, a scale of justice which must always be in balance. You do this for me and I'll do that for you. In reality, there's an ebb and flow of giving and taking between two people. The one with greater capacity gives more until they become depleted, then it's the other person's turn to be generous.

After David died, I needed an embarrassing level of help. But I discovered if I could get really clear about what I needed and ask the right person — someone who could get it done without too much of a stretch — they would deliver almost every time. Everyone likes being a hero. The key is to get crystal clear so you can ask specifically, and the person can feel free to say, "I can or can't do that." It completely debunks the idea that people don't want to give you what you're asking for.

It comes down to, "Can I trust you with me?"
What is my next, best move?
Reflection or structure or action.

First, make clear distinctions and figure out what you want to ask. Be very specific, so that the person you ask can deliver exactly what's needed. Center yourself, then make your request clearly and powerfully, without attachment to the outcome. Whether they say 'Yes' or 'No', be sure they know you are going to be fine.

Second, look at the five areas of affluence (work/business, health, money, relationships and time) to see what request would make the most difference. Get clear before you ask. Start building the muscle, understanding that someone wants to give you what you're asking for, if they can provide it easily.

Who/what do I need for a robust, invigorating social life?

- Drinks

- Eating out

- Music

- Theater

- Museums

- Entertainment

- Family – Mine or David's

- Friends – old and new

Who/what do I need for health?

- Exercise

- Dance

- Movement

- Yoga

- Nutrition

- Hydration

- Sleep

Who/what do I need for business?

- Brainstorming
- Networking
- Referrals
- Funding
- JV Partnerships
- Team

Who/what do I need for financial wellbeing?

- Clients
- Team
- Operations
- Systems

Who/what do I need for self-care and self-expression?

- Walk in nature
- Meditation
- Singing
- Writing poetry
- Taking baths
- Prayer

Finally, ask the right person in the right way to get what you want. The key is to figure out who that person is. Who can deliver what you are asking for? No one, especially widows and widowers, wants to incur a debt they might not be able to fulfill. I discovered that gracious asking and receiving creates an equal exchange with no obligation.

Questions to Ask for a Thriving Network

1. What do I need as a widow on my own that I did not need as a wife with a partner?

2. Are there people I need to disconnect from? Or people I should reach out to?

3. How can I be proactive in nurturing and calling on my networks?

In working with clients, I show them how to assess their networks in all areas of their lives and to identify who is essential to their thriving. If there are gaps—and there are always gaps—I support them in looking for the right people to rise into those roles. Once they know what's missing, it's easy to design a network of people able and eager to deliver anything they might ask.

Ask yourself, "What's the destination? And what strategic actions and connections will get me there?"

One of my most difficult to explain connections is with David's mother, Joyce. Often contentious while we were married, it turned into a treasured, loving relationship after he died. We share our deep grief about the loss of my husband, her son, and I see her at least twice a week. Meanwhile, I am also in a committed relationship with my boyfriend, Wayne. I wrote this poem recently to try to describe the complexity of my ties to my mother-in-law.

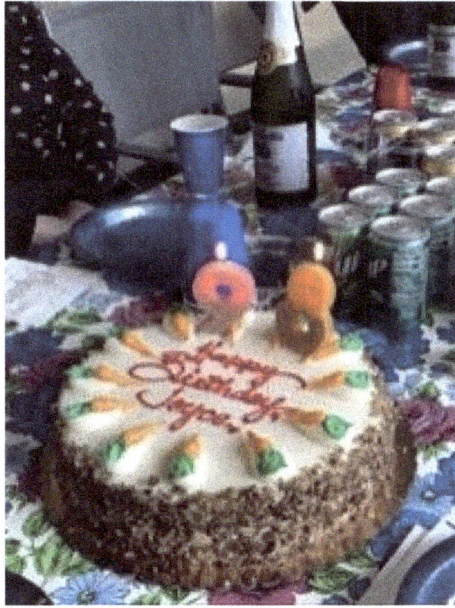

Carrot cake from Veniero's

Her 98th Birthday

Pitched battles when my husband, David, was alive
His mother tugging him,
like a taut rope in a children's game,
Feet braced I, on the other end, his wife.

Hard words, slammed doors, misunderstandings,
For ten years, he took her side,
decades of history in play.
Then the tide turned. In the end our love prevailed,
He and me, a triumph bittersweet.

The man we both loved, was gone.
Leaving us each other, wife and mother,
A promise made.

He always planned extravaganzas on her birthday.
Now it's up to me to transform the celebration,
So much theirs, and make it ours without him,
Sadness into light.

Love came hard between us but it came for us,
since David died, a peculiar gift.

Her 98[th]birthday, a garden party planned by me,
So many things go wrong.
That day the trees are sprayed with pesticides,
Torrential rain, not sun.

Love comes in different packages,
sneaks up unexpectedly,
sweet and sour.

Into the wheelchair, excited, she is ready to go,
Pouring rain, her favorite lavender sweater drenched,
By umbrella dripping,
"Brrr, an icy drop just slid down my neck,"
she shudders and laughs.

Running fast, almost flying,
dodging cracks, uneven sidewalk,
Scared I'll dump her out, she shouts at me, apologizes.
Tells me she's afraid I will go away,
if she gets angry.

When I take her home at six o'clock,
after carrot cake with friends
She says, "I think I love you more than ever before."
I understand completely, thinking, "Yes, me too."

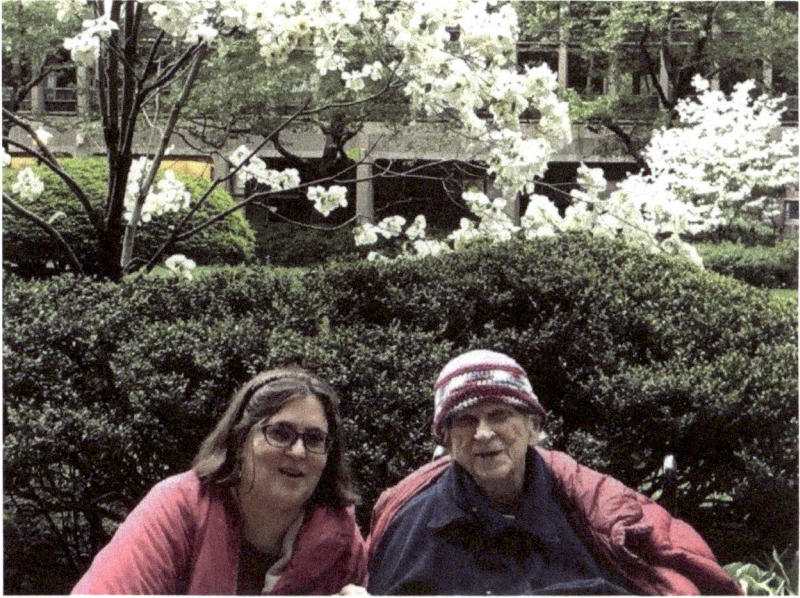

After the rain, the sun came out.

Insights

People who are grieving often feel abandoned by friends and family, whom they thought they could count on, if they are too emotional and difficult to be with. We are all hardwired to fix whatever is hurting the people we love. But grief can't be fixed and it's distressing to witness, helpless to heal their pain.

Action Steps

1. Observe who stuck with you, which family and friends stepped up or stepped back but didn't leave you. What roles do they play in your life? What resources do they provide you, and what additional support might they provide if asked specifically?

2. What kinds of support are missing because some of the people who supported you are gone? Or maybe they passed away. Losing a spouse leaves an enormous hole that your network was never designed to fill. Clearly identify the gaps.

3. Consider who you want in your network. Who can and will deliver on your dreams? Look around for the best people and invite them in proactively.

If you are looking for grief support and tips, subscribe to my free Life After Grief newsletter, delivered to your inbox weekly. https://grief.beehiiv.com

To see more David Beynon Pena artworks for sale, go to https://chairish.com/shop/penafineart

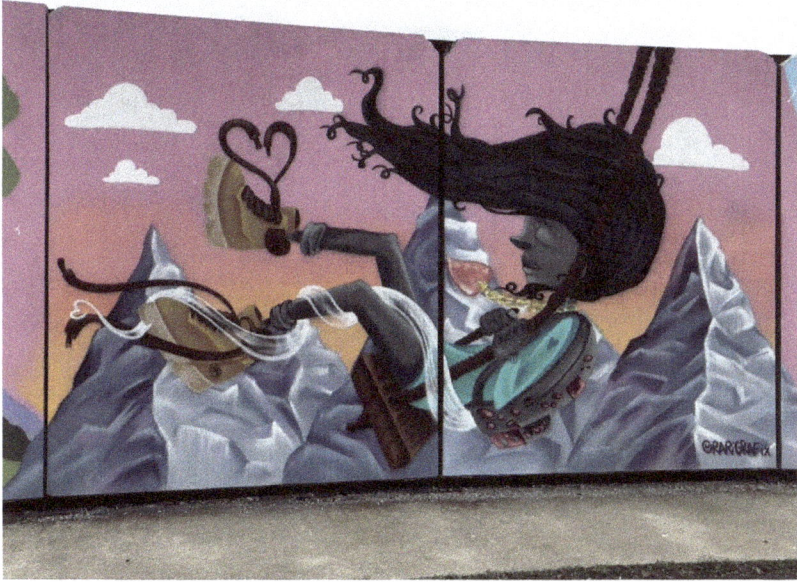

This is one of the scenes in a mural painting called the Wishing Wall in Sleepy Hollow, NY. It was envisioned by members of the community and many people participated in its creation. The idea was to create a visual representation of their dreams for themselves, their families, their community and the world. It's inspiring. I invite you to look it up.

This is often how I felt, kicking my way out of rocky places, lifted up by love.

'You'll Never Walk Alone'

"When you walk through a storm
Hold your head up high
And don't be afraid of the dark

At the end of a storm
There's a golden sky
And the sweet silver song of a lark

Walk on through the wind
Walk on through the rain
Though your dreams be tossed and blown

Walk on, walk on
With hope in your heart
And you'll never walk alone

You'll never walk alone"

Rodgers and Hammerstein
Carousel 1945

I sang the Gerry and the Pacemakers cover version of this song often at open mics that first year, sharing my grief and belief in love itself.

CHAPTER 9

Risking Heartbreak Again For Love

There are 13.7 million widowed persons and 11 million are women. While married, women tend to give up more of their autonomy than men. As widows, they are less likely to make critical compromises. Unwilling to live the rest of my life without love, I was also terrified to risk loving again.

I loved and lived with David for almost half my life. Seeing the breath go out of his body, holding him, was an amazingly intimate, but heartbreaking experience. Afterwards, it was terrifying to open up to the possibility of suffering through that bone-deep pain again. For 25 years, his skin and body were all I knew. Seeking love, wanting to love and be loved again, was natural, but I couldn't imagine any other body than his feeling right next to mine. Amongst the challenges I faced, being willing to open up to joy again was hardest of all. If David wasn't here, it felt wrong to be joyful without him.

The last time I dated was in 1992. That's when I met David, and we were married in October of 1996. It was now 2018, so I was out of practice at dating. But I decided I had to try. I went to listen to live music at a bar. This guy began chatting me up, whining about how awful his ex-wife was. And I'm sitting there thinking, "At what point, do I tell him my husband died quite recently? How fast does that kill the conversation?"

As to the advice I got from friends, it was contradictory, ranging from "I know David would want you to start dating soon," (just four months after he died in 2016), to "That's way too fast," (in 2018). Whenever someone tells you what to do, check to see if their advice is true for you before you follow it. I usually say, "Thank you so much. I'll take that under consideration."

People have lots of ideas about how a widow should act, especially in the area of love. The biggest question is, "When is it acceptable to date, without being judged?"

Initially, even considering love swamped me in grief. The idea of being with anyone but David brought up enormous waves of tears and memories. To risk loving and being loved again, my goal had to be so big that it would make the pain worthwhile. I told myself, "I get to have a second epic love affair in my life." For me, it wasn't enough just to date or to be in the company of men, to not be lonely, missing touch. But the big goal is not the same for everyone, so figuring out what YOU want for yourself is critical to reaching your goal.

I started with a two-year dating plan — to play, doing activities I enjoyed with men who had similar tastes. My only goal, on the first date, was to decide if I wanted a second one. It took six months before I could allow myself to be kissed without having a panic attack. I was not an easy person to date, much less to be with in a relationship.

Online Dating Adventures

With limited capacity to reach out to people, I chose a dating app, Bumble, and started swiping left and right. Online dating seemed like a more efficient way to meet the right men at a time when I had little energy to spare and needed to screen out any who might drain me further. I needed to find someone who was emotionally available, responsible for themselves and comfortable with their own mortality.

The online dating world was crazy. I flipped through dozens of profiles with endless photos of men holding fish, in front of sports cars, suggestive shots taken in a bathroom, in front of an unmade bed, even one bare-chested man with a Mother tattoo. There were blurry photos. Some men wrote nothing. Others tried to be sarcastic or witty or whiny.

I quickly determined I had no interest in men who were looking at me to 'complete' them. I wanted each person to bring their own 100%. I looked for men who tried to say something about themselves with words. My screening process was fierce. It was mostly quick swipes to the left, eliminating 90% of the possibilities.

The first person I saw on Bumble that I thought was cool was a bagpipe player for the NFL. It was such a quirky job, intriguing. I wrote, "I'd really love to meet you. This is my first time." He got rid of me so fast!

At the start, I made many mistakes. I had a little pewter unicorn that I put on my profile and I started getting all these suggestive, explicitly sexual messages. I did not realize that a unicorn in online dating speak is not a mythological creature from a child's tale. My girlfriend called me seven times to say, "Get that unicorn off your profile!"

At first, I only liked people who were four hours away from me, impossible to meet in person. A clue that I was getting closer to ready was when I began liking men who lived close enough to actually go on a date.

When I started dating, my profile focused on activities I wanted to do with a man. I was trying to attract men who liked to do what I enjoyed myself, with the thought that "Even if there isn't a lot of chemistry, we'd both have fun." Intimacy was not even on the table.

Setting Up a Winning Profile

I described myself as clearly as I could, offering specific likes and dislikes. "I prefer rocky beaches to sandy ones." So, if the Jersey Shore is your favorite vacation spot, not my guy. I wanted people to make a choice, "Yes, that's a person for me" or "No, she's not for me." If they didn't want to date a widow, I encouraged them to swipe left. I tweaked photos and words until I started getting responses from men I found interesting and wanted to meet. My screening process was also about discovering what kind of man I liked, since I no longer knew. By the time I went on my first date, my level of clarity was so specific, I didn't have a single, awful dating experience.

Clarity is essential, because until you figure out what you want, you're not going to get it. When I started dating, I read multiple profiles and looked at endless photos to figure out what characteristics I was looking for, so that I would recognize the right person when they showed up. And I worked to describe myself so clearly that if they were looking for me, they could find me.

Some people have told me they don't think it should be necessary to offer such a clear profile description of themselves. "If they know me, they should just know what I want." That's ridiculous. Many profiles are written to describe the lifestyle they want with that future person, instead of asking who you are, who they are and whether you will like each other's company. And it probably means you're not going to get whoever it is you want.

Writing and tweaking your profile and photos is a powerful way to discover who you are now, at a time of massive change, while also letting potential dates know what your interests are and what you like to do. Watching the kind of men you get with each profile change you make is also a valuable tool to clarify who you are now, and what you want. I didn't worry about attracting lots of men, their height, weight or even their bank account during my preliminary screening process. At the end of this dating journey, I wanted to find one man who wanted me, exactly as I was.

For me, the desire for a second epic love affair in my life was enough to transition through barrier after barrier, from having another man's arm around my waist, to being kissed even when it sparked panic attacks, to the ever-present judgmental questioning, "David was the love of my life. How dare I desire another one?! But I did.

Seeking to deter anyone who wasn't for me, I had three criteria which were deal breakers: 1) no smokers, 2) no Trump people, and 3) must love music. I was looking for men who shared my values, with whom I could feel safe at a time when I was so vulnerable. I wanted men to go out with, to keep pushing my own edges, who liked the same kinds of things that I liked. I figured once we met, I could find out if there was more connection between us. It was a beginning, not a fast track to marriage, short-term intimacy or a committed relationship. I was not ready... yet.

Self-expression heals me and helps me feel whole. I write poetry to try to make sense of things, like "Desire Clear as Mud", exploring the confusion of love, lust, longing and loss. Perhaps you may see yourself here too.

Desire Clear as Mud

Clear as mud,
what I want, what you want, who I am.
Settled, steeped, stuck
In the mud.

Your courting words confuse me –
beautiful, gorgeous, honey –
and offend me,
feeling not exactly true.

My radar for lies acute,
like barnacle tentacles waving,
testing the environment.
unsure of what I feel.

You don't know me, but neither do I,
tapping along blindly, testing the edges
of my widow's cage.

Assumptions, agreements, obligations…
Love delighted and bound me
to his desire, my desire, our desires
until I no longer know what is true.

Autonomy is sweet and bitter,
Alone, I choose, I alone
from my old and my new longings,
No 'right' desires, simply mine.

Easier than 'Yes" is "No,"
digging for answers, clear as mud.

Negative space reveals
my 'not' desires made clear.

Like building a sandcastle on the beach,
structural with sand, fluid with seawater,
magic imagined, no two the same
Like me and you.

Made and destroyed by the ocean, by a child,
wrecked by my grief, dancing in the street,
feeling longing and lust, while kisses cause panic,
my turned cheek of avoidance, and so it goes.

As a clam,
mud's a fine place to be,
tunneling down to safe,
squirting up, "I am here."

But I am not a clam.
I know mud can be shaped into anything.

Finding Wayne on Bumble

When I had my first Bumble date on Sunday, July 1st, 2018, I had not dated since 1992. His name was Wayne, and I responded to his note with, "It's a hot day, so I'm going to a movie" (naming two possibilities). "Why don't we get together one day?" His answer, "Let's go to Jurassic World," one of the movies I suggested, "and let's have 'one day' be today." Intrigued, I said "Yes."

I was so torn, both excited and terrified. I couldn't imagine being with another man. It felt like betraying David, to desire love again. But I was unwilling to live out the rest of my life alone.

On the way to our first date, Wayne listened to one of my guest podcasts. One of the characteristics which drew me to him from the start was that he listened to me, my real experience as a widow, without making assumptions.

When Wayne and I started dating, we took turns deciding what to do and each date was about learning more about each other. His first date plan was to go to Whole Foods and alternate choosing food for a picnic, and with each choice, we had to say why. Then we took our picnic, walked down to the WW II East Coast Memorial benches, opposite the Statue of Liberty, to eat, talk and laugh. My first date was a graffiti mural crawl in East Harlem, starting at 96th Street and Park, wandering all the way up to 125th Street. Then we went and listened to a blues band at Gin Fizz on Lenox Avenue in Harlem. We both love exploring New York City on foot.

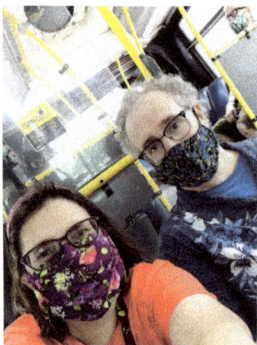

A pandemic bus date

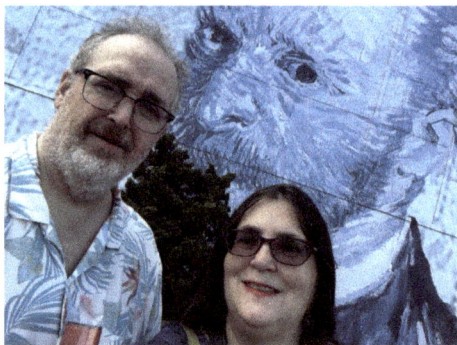

Immersive Van Gogh art date

Prioritizing Clear, Honest Communication

We also found a way to deal with my emotional ups and downs. Our only agreement was that I would communicate, "This is what's going on with me," without blaming him or shaming myself for my feelings. Whether I was happy, sad, angry or afraid, Wayne let me be. I was a hot mess and this one man kept showing up.

David, my husband, was the only one to touch me for 25 years. Now I couldn't trust my own chemistry, as touch sparked both desire and revulsion.

When I experienced this body reaction, I had to ask myself, "Is it me? Is it him? Or is it us?" Once I had my answer, I then knew my next best action to take. If it was me, I had to handle my emotions responsibly and clean up any miscommunications. If it was him, I had to tell him what was not working for me. If it was us, we needed to solve the issue together.

These distinctions made such a difference to the foundation of clear communication that we built together. I told him, "Don't try to fix me. There's nothing wrong with me. I may cry but I'm not broken." Eventually, I was able to be kissed without a going into a panic attack.

Wayne just kept getting it right. I would burst into tears and say, "It's this anniversary. I'm sorry I'm acting so weird." And he'd say, "I don't mind that you're weird." He told me what a big relief it was to know how to support me.

Often I sent mixed messages, but still Wayne hung in there. In October, I told him not to contact me until January when all my difficult anniversaries were over. Then I invited him to meet my mother at MOMA for my cousin's movie premiere. He must have been getting whiplash trying to follow my moods.

The moment I truly fell in love with Wayne was when we were meant to get together for a date, and it turned out to be on an anniversary I'd forgotten, so I was crying all day. I was looking forward to getting together for our date, but I was a hot mess. I thought, "What to do? Do I cancel? It isn't his fault I'm like this."

In the end, I decided he was an adult who could decide for himself, so I called and told him, "I have been crying all day and I want to see you, but I have no idea how I'm going to be. It's your choice. We can reschedule if you're not up for this today." He chose to see me anyway, just as I was, even if I wept.

Daring Intimacy in Tarrytown

I met Wayne on July 1st 2018 and by Christmas, we decided we wanted to move in together. But we had never been intimate. And I did not know if I could get through my tears and fears.

We both knew we would need to deepen our relationship and have sex or part ways. So we decided to go away together for the weekend to a hotel in Tarrytown. The only rule was one room, one bed. We made no other promises.

Wayne had been patient for six months, and as long as he could see that I was trying, he could continue being patient. But we had to communicate everything for it to work. For both of us, the goal was to get to the other side of my heartbroken messiness to fully realize love. I wasn't willing to live without intimate love and he wasn't willing to give me up without a fight.

I packed a pair of red-and-white spotted Navy pajamas, two negligees and hoped to get to naked by the end. When I faced Wayne in that hotel room, after changing into my pajamas in the bathroom, I stood before him, raised my arms shyly and said, "Is this okay?" My body was not the same as it was in 1992. I didn't feel as confident as I did back then.

I'd heard it was normal for a widow to cry having sex for the first time after the death of a spouse, so I thought I would have one good hard cry and be done. But I ended up crying, off and on, through the entire weekend.

It required pressing up against deep fears of being touched intimately, embarrassment about my no longer young body, and feelings of guilt about moving on, over and over again. Every time I said 'Stop!' or went into a panic attack, he stopped. We took the time I needed to calm myself, then pressed on again.

"If you're willing to be that brave," he told me, "I can be that patient." It was very tough. Lots of tears, but now we live together.

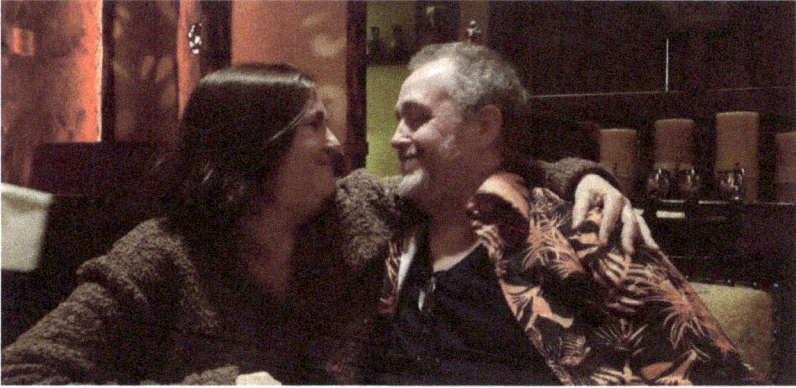

About to kiss in Vegas, happy to be together (Photo by Boz)

When Wayne Moved In

My husband David was a professional artist whose 39-year legacy of art occupies every corner of the apartment. So anyone who wants to be with me has to be okay with that reality.

When Wayne agreed to move in with me, we talked about making changes to help him feel at home. But I was not prepared for my reaction that first day, when he walked in, looked around and asked, "OK, now what changes are we going to make?"

I freaked out, saying, "You are all the change I can handle!" Then, after my outburst, we moved the furniture around to create a more comfortable living space for the two of us, and to shake off some of my memories of living in the same apartment with David.

SIDE NOTE TO READER: this chapter describes <u>my</u> path back to love. You may or may not want that. Love can take many forms – self-love, friendship, companionship, whatever you desire for yourself. Every person's journey through grief is their own. I chose to risk another intimate love when I was ready (or rather willing to be ready). Find out what <u>you</u> want and then take your first step in that direction.

Insight

Hearts are tender but resilient. After losing a loved one to death, divorce or breakup, we hurt. It's tempting to close down and avoid taking that risk again. But if you do, you miss one of life's greatest adventures. Your life and your choice. The journey is hard, but I swear it's worth it, opening up to love and be loved again.

Action Steps

1. Remember that the past does not predict the future. Remember that no matter what your previous experience of love, you are worthy to love and be loved, exactly as you are. Start with one date, knowing any connection takes practice if you're rusty.

2. Get clear on who you are and what activities you like, so that you can invite another person who enjoys the same to play with you. Be specific. Define your non-negotiable dealbreakers to allow potential dates to say, 'No,' if you are not their person. Narrow the field to the right possibilities.

3. Watch the results you get and use the information to make even more distinctions about who and what you truly desire. I found my second true love for a lifetime in six months. It wasn't easy. But love is worth fighting for. In any form that pleases you.

RESOURCES

If you are looking for grief support and tips, subscribe to my
free Life After Grief newsletter, delivered to your
inbox weekly. https://grief.beehiiv.com

To see more David Beynon Pena artworks for sale, go to
https://chairish.com/shop/penafineart

ACKNOWLEDGEMENTS

First and foremost, I want to thank my mother and editor, Anne White, for her invaluable and dedicated help in making this dream a reality, with multiple rounds of editing, encouragement, straight talk and love. I truly could not have finished this without you.

To my boyfriend, Wayne Hacker, for taking a chance on me when I was a hot mess and for every day since, I love you. You saw me truly from the start.

To my best friend, Roberta Moss, thank you for being there for me through thick and thin. I love you.

To my dear friend, Susie Ward, for telling me that last day, as I held David in my arms after he left me, that I didn't have to rush to let the rest of the world in.

To Camille Nisich, for over 5 + years of business accountability and friendship, advancing our business goals, I am grateful. You are my M-F, 7-8 am rock.

To my friend, Betsy Cox Murphy, for reading my words and offering exactly the help I needed at an especially tough moment. You are wonderful.

To Eric Michaelson, for being my friend after David died, helping me clear and close out the studio, and especially for letting me be sad without running away, I am so grateful. It would been so much harder without you.

To Joyce Jessie Pena, for all the years with and without David and the tears we've shared since he died. I love you, and am glad to have you in my life.

To David Beynon Pena, with gratitude for our life together and for my journey on alone, the crucible which turned me into Bad Widow.

To my family, David's family and the friends who care about me, I love you and am grateful for all the ways you've supported me these last years.

To Emi Kirschner, for believing in me even when I doubted myself, intuitive business expertise and for helping me keep going.

To Bernadette Pleasant and Maurya Sullivan, our fearless leaders, and my WomanSpeak Circle, thank you for shared stories, powerful feedback and a loving, safe space to be fully myself.

To my teacher, Leslie Berliant, and my fellow Writing from the Deep Voice participants, thank you for reminding me to keep the stories deeply personal when I feared to dive deep.

To D'Ambrose Boyd and the family of my heart at Singers Space Open Mic, I love you. You and the music kept me whole. D'Ambrose, your hugs when I was starved for human touch meant everything to me.

To Bill Buschel and the Hudson Valley Writers Center Open Mic regulars, who witnessed my words and singing without judgement, even the sad ones. Thank you for your kind words and caring.

To The Artists Fellowship Board, which provided financial and emotional support to sustain me, especially Everett and Peggy Kinstler, Charlie Yoder, Babette Bloch and Marc Mellon, and Morton Kaish.

To Brendan Rooney, for endless kindness, robust support, and putting me back on solid ground.

To Yolanda Langlois, thank you always for your compassion and understanding after David died, and for giving me the time I needed to get back on my feet.

To Iman and Afrin Khan, and the Red Elephant Herd, everyone needs a business family to stand for them and you are one of mine.

To Marcus Bell, Peaches Udoma and the Wealth & Impact Bootcamp participants, thank you for your insights and feedback which helped me focus and accelerated my progress in getting this book done.

To everyone else who supported me along the way, because writing a book takes a village, I appreciate you.

To all the podcast, radio show and summit hosts who invited me to be a guest on their platforms and share my story and resources to move through grief more peacefully and effectively with their audiences, thank you very much.

Dragons Fly

"They fly. The dragons fly. Did you see them?" the small boy asked, tugging at his grandmother's sleeve.

She looked at him blankly. She saw nothing. Most adults lose the magic in the world when they grow up. They forget how, with all that focusing on practical things. "Stop making things up. What an imagination you have, child."

He continued to gaze skyward at them flying, each colored according to their nature: scarlet fire dragons with licks and lashes of flame escaping their form, ultramarine water dragons pregnant with drops of clear, lifegiving aqua, ephemeral air dragons, seen only against the clouds in all colors of the rainbow and burnt umber earth dragons, deeply connected to the crystals they nurture under the earth.

The dragons delighted in his rapt attention, dancing in the sky for him and the fire dragon flamed great gouts of yellow-red-brown as he flew, bursting beauteous destruction, revelation and reincarnation from his gaping maw. But only the child saw and he was not afraid. He was a bit magical himself, after all.

Alison Pena

As September 10, 2024 will be eight years since David died, sometimes I escape into writing about magic. Enjoy!

Life is short. I invite you to live yours fully and joyfully.

www.ingramcontent.com/pod-product-compliance
Lightning Source LLC
Chambersburg PA
CBHW042248040426
42336CB00043B/3362